Yoga for Kids:

The Ultimate Guide to Yoga for Bend, Breathe, and Grow with Empowering Children through Mindfulness, Flexibility, and Fun with Yoga

Laura Trenaman

Table of Contents

Introduction

In the hustle and bustle of today's fast-paced world, where screens dominate and schedules are packed, the need for holistic well-being for our children has never been more critical. As parents, educators, and caregivers, we are on a quest to provide the next generation with tools to navigate life's challenges while fostering resilience, self-awareness, and a strong sense of self.

Enter the world of "Yoga for Kids: The Ultimate Guide to Yoga for Bend, Breathe, and Grow." This comprehensive guide is a heartfelt invitation to embark on a transformative journey with your children—one that seamlessly integrates the ancient wisdom of yoga into the vibrant tapestry of modern childhood. It's not just about teaching kids to touch their toes; it's about empowering them to touch the depths of their inner resilience, strength, and joy.

Mindfulness, Flexibility, and Fun

In these pages, you will discover more than just a collection of yoga poses for kids. You will find a treasure trove of mindful practices, breathing exercises, and playful activities designed to nurture the mind, body, and spirit of your young ones. Yoga becomes a powerful vehicle for instilling qualities like focus, patience, and compassion, all while encouraging physical strength and flexibility.

Each chapter unfolds a new dimension of the yoga experience, offering age-appropriate guidance for different stages of childhood. From the lively and imaginative sessions suited for energetic toddlers to the more focused and contemplative practices for older kids, "Yoga for Kids" adapts to the unique needs of your child's developmental journey.

Empowering Children through Yoga

Beyond the physical postures, this guide delves into the heart of what makes yoga a transformative practice—self-discovery, self-expression, and self-empowerment. Through carefully crafted sequences, storytelling, and interactive exercises, children learn not only to move their bodies but also to tune in to their emotions, thoughts, and the world around them. The mat becomes a magical space where they can explore, express, and embrace the full spectrum of their being.

The benefits extend far beyond the mat. As children cultivate mindfulness and flexibility in a joyful and non-competitive environment, they carry these skills into their daily lives. The tools acquired through yoga become lifelong companions, assisting them in facing challenges, building resilience, and nurturing a positive relationship with their bodies and minds.

A Journey of Connection

This book is not just a guide for children but an invitation for adults to connect with the young ones in their lives on a deeper level. Through shared yoga experiences, whether as a family or in a classroom setting, relationships are strengthened, and communication deepens. "Yoga for Kids" offers a bridge between generations, creating moments of joy, laughter, and connection that resonate far beyond the physical practice.

So, join us on this extraordinary journey of bending, breathing, and growing—a journey that goes beyond the yoga mat and into the hearts of the children we cherish. Let's empower the next generation to face life's challenges with grace, cultivate inner strength, and embark on a lifelong adventure of well-being and self-discovery. Welcome to "Yoga for

Kids"—where mindfulness meets playfulness, flexibility meets resilience, and every breath is an opportunity to grow.

Welcome to the World of Kids' Yoga

In the magical realm where imagination intertwines with movement, and curiosity dances with breath, we welcome you to the enchanting world of Kids' Yoga. This is a space where the vibrant energy of childhood converges with the ancient wisdom of yoga, creating a harmonious symphony of joy, discovery, and growth.

Embarking on a Journey of Playful Exploration

In this world, every yoga mat becomes a portal to adventure. Picture toddlers giggling like little raindrops, mimicking frogs and butterflies, their bodies bending and stretching in delightful sync. Visualize older children striking warrior poses with determination, their minds focused and their hearts open. Kids' Yoga is more than just a physical activity; it's a journey of playful exploration that nurtures the holistic development of our young ones.

Where Mindfulness Meets Playfulness

Kids' Yoga is a celebration of mindfulness and playfulness coexisting in perfect harmony. It's about introducing children to the transformative power of breath, teaching them to be present in each moment. Yet, it's also a world where the mat transforms into a spaceship, and traditional poses become characters in an unfolding story. As children move and breathe, they learn to navigate the delicate balance between focus and fun, mindfulness and imagination.

Fostering a Lifelong Love for Health and Well-being

Step into this world, and you'll witness the seeds of a lifelong love for health and well-being being sown. Kids' Yoga goes beyond the mat, instilling in children a sense of body awareness, promoting flexibility, and cultivating a positive relationship with physical activity. Through the playful integration of yoga philosophy, children learn valuable life skills such as patience, resilience, and empathy, setting the stage for a journey of self-discovery and empowerment.

Connecting Hearts, Strengthening Bonds

But it's not just about individual growth; it's about connection. Kids' Yoga becomes a shared experience, a bond between caregivers, educators, and the little ones in their care. Together, they embark on a journey that transcends the boundaries of age and generation, creating moments of laughter, joy, and understanding. Through shared breaths and synchronized movements, hearts connect, fostering a sense of community and support.

A World Where Every Child Shines

In the world of Kids' Yoga, every child is a shining star. Regardless of ability or background, each young yogi is encouraged to express themselves authentically, embrace their uniqueness, and discover the strength that resides within them. It's a world that celebrates diversity, encourages self-love, and nurtures a sense of belonging—a world where every child is seen, heard, and valued.

So, step onto the mat, open your heart to the possibilities that unfold, and let the journey begin. Welcome to the World of Kids' Yoga, where movement is a celebration, breath is a friend, and every child is a radiant beacon of potential.

The Benefits of Yoga for Children

In a world that often moves at a whirlwind pace, introducing children to the ancient practice of yoga can be a transformative gift. Beyond its reputation as a physical exercise, yoga for children offers a myriad of holistic benefits that extend to their mental, emotional, and social well-being. Here are some of the remarkable advantages:

1. **Physical Well-being:**

Yoga poses for children promote flexibility, strength, and balance. As they engage in various postures, their bodies develop awareness, coordination, and improved motor skills. Regular practice contributes to a healthy, active lifestyle, laying the foundation for a lifetime of physical well-being.

2.   Emotional Regulation:

Yoga encourages children to explore and understand their emotions. Through mindful breathing and movement, they learn to identify and manage stress, anxiety, and frustration. The practice provides a safe space for emotional expression, fostering emotional intelligence and resilience.

3.   Enhanced Concentration:

The art of focused breathing and mindful movement in yoga helps improve attention span and concentration. As children learn to be present in the moment, they develop the capacity to stay focused, both in the classroom and in their daily activities.

4.   Stress Reduction:

In a world filled with stimuli, children are not immune to stress. Yoga offers them tools to navigate and alleviate stress. Simple breathing exercises and relaxation techniques empower children to create a sense of calm, promoting mental clarity and emotional well-being.

5.   Boosted Self-Esteem:

Yoga is a non-competitive practice that encourages self-acceptance and self-expression. As children achieve new poses and milestones, they experience a sense of accomplishment that contributes to a positive self-image and boosts self-esteem.

6. Social Interaction:

Participating in group yoga classes fosters a sense of community and social connection. Children learn to respect others' space, listen actively, and cooperate in a supportive environment. These social skills extend beyond the mat into various aspects of their lives.

7. Mind-Body Connection:

Yoga emphasizes the integration of mind and body. By connecting breath with movement, children develop a heightened awareness of their bodies. This mind-body connection lays the groundwork for a positive relationship with physical activity and self-care.

8. Improved Sleep Patterns:

The calming effects of yoga, especially relaxation techniques and gentle stretches, contribute to improved sleep quality. Establishing a bedtime yoga routine can be particularly beneficial, helping children unwind and prepare for a restful night's sleep.

9.   Cultivation of Mindfulness:

Mindfulness, the practice of being fully present, is a cornerstone of yoga. Children learn to observe their thoughts and sensations without judgment. This skill enhances their ability to navigate challenges with a clear mind and a centered presence.

10. Lifelong Healthy Habits:

Introducing children to yoga instills healthy habits early in life. The positive experiences on the mat create a foundation for a lifelong appreciation of movement, mindfulness, and self-care, contributing to their overall well-being into adulthood.

In essence, yoga for children is a holistic and empowering practice that transcends the physical, offering tools for navigating the complexities of growing up with resilience, self-awareness, and a joyful heart.

Chapter 1: Understanding the Basics

In the journey of introducing children to the transformative world of yoga, it's essential to start with a solid foundation. This chapter lays the groundwork by delving into the fundamental aspects of kids' yoga, offering insights into its origins, guiding principles, and unique considerations when teaching yoga to children.

1. The Roots of Kids' Yoga: A Brief History

Explore the historical roots of yoga and its evolution into a practice tailored specifically for children. From ancient yogic traditions to the contemporary embrace of kids' yoga, understanding its origins provides context for the richness and adaptability of this age-old practice.

2. The Core Principles of Kids' Yoga

Examine the core principles that form the heart of kids' yoga. From cultivating mindfulness and promoting self-expression to fostering a non-competitive and inclusive environment, these principles guide both practitioners and instructors in creating a positive and nurturing space for children to explore and grow.

3. Adapting Yoga for Different Age Groups

Children of different ages have unique needs, attention spans, and physical abilities. Learn how to tailor yoga sessions to suit specific age groups, ensuring that the practices are both engaging and developmentally appropriate. This section provides practical insights and age-specific considerations for effective teaching.

4. Creating a Safe and Supportive Environment

Safety is paramount in kids' yoga. Discover the importance of creating a safe and supportive environment for children to explore and express themselves. From proper mat placement to effective communication techniques, this section offers valuable tips on fostering a space where children feel secure and encouraged.

5. The Art of Storytelling in Kids' Yoga

One of the enchanting aspects of kids' yoga is the incorporation of storytelling. Understand how the art of storytelling enhances engagement, captivates young minds, and seamlessly weaves yoga poses into imaginative narratives. Learn techniques for crafting compelling stories that inspire movement and mindfulness.

6. Incorporating Playfulness into Practice

Kids thrive on play, and incorporating playfulness into yoga sessions can make the practice both enjoyable and effective. Explore creative and playful approaches to teaching yoga poses, breathing exercises, and mindfulness activities. This section provides a toolbox of ideas to infuse joy into every yoga session.

7. Tools and Props for Kids' Yoga

Introduce a variety of tools and props that can enhance the kids' yoga experience. From colorful mats and props to visual aids, discover how these elements can add an extra layer of engagement and excitement, making the practice more dynamic and enjoyable for children.

By delving into the basics of kids' yoga, this chapter sets the stage for a holistic exploration of the practice. As we understand its roots, principles, and unique considerations, we pave the way for a journey that is not only enriching and educational but also filled with the joy and wonder that children bring to every yoga session.

1.1 What is Yoga?

At its essence, yoga is a holistic practice that unites the mind, body, and spirit, fostering a harmonious balance between these interconnected facets of our being. Rooted in ancient Indian philosophy, yoga transcends a mere physical exercise regimen; it is a journey of self-discovery, self-discipline, and spiritual exploration.

1. Physical Practice:

Yoga often begins as a physical practice, involving a series of postures or poses known as "asanas." These asanas promote flexibility, strength, and balance, enhancing overall physical well-being. The physical aspect of yoga is a gateway, inviting individuals to connect with their bodies and cultivate a heightened awareness of movement and breath.

2.   Breath Awareness:

Central to yoga is the art of mindful breathing, known as "pranayama." Breath is considered a bridge between the body and the mind, and conscious breath awareness serves as a powerful tool for calming the mind, reducing stress, and promoting mental clarity. In yoga, the breath is often synchronized with movement to create a fluid and meditative practice.

3.   Meditation and Mindfulness:

Beyond the physical postures, yoga incorporates meditation and mindfulness practices. These techniques encourage individuals to turn their attention inward, observing thoughts and sensations without judgment. Through regular meditation, practitioners develop a profound sense of presence and self-awareness.

4.   Philosophy and Ethics:

Yoga is grounded in a rich philosophical tradition outlined in ancient texts like the Yoga Sutras of Patanjali. These teachings provide ethical guidelines for living a meaningful and purposeful life, emphasizing virtues such as compassion, truthfulness, and non-attachment. The philosophical aspect of yoga extends beyond the mat, influencing one's approach to daily life.

5.   Union and Connection:

The word "yoga" itself means union, signifying the integration of the individual self with the universal consciousness. This union extends to the interconnectedness of all living beings and the harmonious relationship between humans and the natural world. Yoga fosters a sense of connection, compassion, and unity.

6.   Spiritual Exploration:

For many, yoga is a spiritual practice that transcends religious boundaries. It provides a space for individuals to explore their spiritual dimensions, connect with a higher consciousness, or deepen their understanding of their own existence. Yoga invites a journey inward, encouraging self-reflection and spiritual growth.

7.   Personal Transformation:

Ultimately, yoga is a path of personal transformation. As individuals engage in the practice over time, they may experience a profound shift in their physical health, mental clarity, emotional well-being, and overall outlook on life. Yoga becomes a lifestyle, influencing choices and behaviors beyond the confines of the yoga mat.

In its entirety, yoga is a holistic system that addresses the multifaceted nature of human existence. Whether approached as a physical exercise, a mindfulness practice, or a spiritual journey, yoga offers a versatile and inclusive path toward self-discovery, well-being, and the realization of our interconnectedness with the world around us.

1.2 How Kids Benefit from Yoga

In a world brimming with constant stimuli and demands, introducing children to the practice of yoga can be a transformative and empowering gift. Beyond its stereotypical association with flexibility and physical postures, kids' yoga offers a holistic approach to well-being that nurtures not only the body but also the mind and spirit. Let's delve into the multifaceted benefits that children reap from embracing the practice of yoga.

1. **Physical Well-being:**

At its core, yoga for kids is a delightful exploration of movement. Through a series of age-appropriate poses and activities, children develop flexibility, strength, and coordination. The physical aspect of yoga is not about competition or perfection; it's about embracing one's own body, fostering a positive relationship with physical activity, and laying the foundation for a healthy, active lifestyle.

2. **Emotional Regulation:**

One of the most profound gifts that yoga bestows upon children is the ability to understand and regulate their emotions. In the safe and supportive environment of a yoga class, kids learn to navigate the landscape of their feelings. Mindful breathing exercises and guided meditations provide them with tools to manage stress, anxiety, and frustration, promoting emotional intelligence and resilience.

3.   Improved Concentration and Focus:

In an age of constant distractions, cultivating focus is a valuable skill for children. The practice of yoga encourages mindful concentration as they engage in various poses, breathing exercises, and relaxation techniques. Over time, this enhanced focus translates into improved attention spans, both in the classroom and in their everyday activities.

4.   Stress Reduction:

Children, like adults, experience stress, and yoga provides a sanctuary for them to release and manage it. Simple breathing exercises and relaxation techniques become powerful tools for young minds, allowing them to unwind and find moments of calm amidst the busyness of their lives. Yoga becomes a refuge where stress dissipates, and a sense of peace prevails.

5.   Boosted Self-Esteem:

In the non-competitive environment of kids' yoga, each child is encouraged to embrace their unique abilities and challenges. As they successfully navigate through poses and activities, a sense of accomplishment emerges, contributing to a positive self-image and boosted self-esteem. Yoga becomes a journey of self-discovery and self-acceptance.

6. Social Interaction and Cooperation:

Participating in group yoga classes fosters a sense of community and social connection. Children learn to respect one another's space, listen actively, and cooperate in a supportive environment. These social skills extend beyond the yoga mat, influencing their interactions with peers and contributing to a positive social outlook.

7. Mind-Body Connection:

Yoga emphasizes the integration of mind and body. Children develop a heightened awareness of their bodies, understanding how movement and breath are intricately connected. This mind-body connection is not only beneficial for physical health but also lays the groundwork for a positive relationship with their bodies and a sense of agency over their well-being.

8. Cultivation of Mindfulness:

Mindfulness, the practice of being fully present in the moment, is a cornerstone of yoga. Through guided exercises and activities, children learn to observe their thoughts and sensations without judgment. This skill becomes a valuable asset as they navigate the challenges of growing up, fostering a sense of clarity and presence in their daily lives.

9. **Improved Sleep Patterns**:

The calming effects of yoga, especially relaxation techniques and gentle stretches, contribute to improved sleep quality. Establishing a bedtime yoga routine can be particularly beneficial, helping children unwind and transition into a restful night's sleep. Adequate, quality sleep is crucial for their overall health and well-being.

10. **Lifelong Healthy Habits:**

Introducing children to yoga at a young age sets the stage for lifelong healthy habits. The positive experiences on the mat create a foundation for an appreciation of movement, mindfulness, and self-care. The habits cultivated in yoga become intrinsic parts of their identity, influencing their choices and behaviors well into adulthood.

In essence, yoga for kids is not just a physical activity; it's a holistic and empowering practice that nurtures the development of the whole child—physically, emotionally, and socially. As children bend and breathe on their yoga mats, they are not only cultivating flexibility in their bodies but also in their hearts and minds. The transformative benefits of yoga ripple through their lives, equipping them with invaluable tools for navigating the challenges of childhood and beyond. It's a journey of self-discovery, resilience, and joy—a journey where each breath becomes an opportunity to grow.

1.3 Getting Started: Setting the Foundation

Embarking on the journey of introducing children to the enriching world of yoga begins with laying a solid foundation. In this initial phase, our focus is on creating an environment that fosters curiosity, joy, and a sense of exploration. Let's delve into the essential steps for getting started and setting the stage for a positive and transformative kids' yoga experience.

1. Create a Welcoming Space:

Begin by establishing a physical environment that is inviting and conducive to the practice of yoga. Whether it's a dedicated space at home, a corner in a classroom, or a community center, make it colorful and comfortable. Use vibrant mats, cushions, and props to create an atmosphere that sparks interest and excitement.

2. Embrace Playfulness:

Kids thrive on play, and incorporating playfulness into the yoga sessions is key. Infuse elements of imagination, storytelling, and creativity into the practice. Allow room for laughter, spontaneity, and exploration. When yoga feels like play, children are more likely to engage wholeheartedly.

3.   Establish Clear Expectations:

Communicate clear and simple expectations to the children before each session. Let them know that yoga is a time for movement, mindfulness, and fun. Emphasize the importance of respecting one another's space, listening actively, and participating with an open heart. Clear expectations create a sense of structure and safety.

4.   Choose Age-Appropriate Activities:

Recognize the diverse developmental stages of the children you are working with and tailor activities accordingly. Younger children may enjoy playful animal poses and interactive games, while older children may engage in more structured sequences and mindfulness exercises. Adapting to their age ensures that the activities are engaging and accessible.

5.   Introduce Mindful Breathing:

Mindful breathing is a fundamental aspect of yoga. Begin each session with simple breathing exercises that capture the children's attention. Explore techniques like "balloon breaths" or "flower breaths" that make breath awareness playful and relatable. These exercises lay the groundwork for cultivating focus and relaxation.

6. Incorporate Music and Movement:

Harness the power of music to enhance the yoga experience. Integrate rhythmic tunes that correspond to the flow of poses or create a calming atmosphere during relaxation. Encourage expressive movement, allowing children to interpret the music through their own unique expressions of yoga poses.

7. Foster Inclusivity:

Yoga is for everyone, regardless of ability or background. Foster inclusivity by offering modifications for different skill levels and ensuring that activities are accessible to all children. Celebrate diversity, and create an atmosphere where each child feels valued and included.

8. Lead by Example:

As the facilitator, embody the spirit of yoga by leading with enthusiasm, compassion, and a sense of wonder. Demonstrate poses with joy, share your own mindfulness practices, and express genuine curiosity about the children's experiences. Your authentic engagement sets a positive tone for the entire group.

9. Encourage Self-Expression:

Create opportunities for children to express themselves through movement and creativity. Allow them to choose poses, express how a particular pose makes them feel, or contribute ideas to the storytelling component of the session. Encouraging self-expression fosters a sense of autonomy and empowerment.

10. Reflect and Adapt:

After each session, take a moment to reflect on what worked well and what might be adapted for future sessions. Be open to feedback from the children, caregivers, or educators involved. The ability to reflect and adapt ensures that the kids' yoga experience remains dynamic and responsive to the evolving needs of the participants.

By taking these foundational steps, you're not only introducing children to the physical aspects of yoga but also cultivating an environment that nurtures their curiosity, creativity, and well-being. This initial phase is a doorway into a world where each child can embark on a journey of self-discovery, resilience, and joy through the practice of yoga. As you set the foundation, remember that the beauty of kids' yoga lies in the simplicity of the present moment and the boundless potential it holds for growth and exploration.

Chapter 2: Yoga Poses for Kids

In the enchanting world of kids' yoga, the introduction of yoga poses becomes a gateway to discovery, imagination, and physical well-being. This chapter invites children and their facilitators to embark on a playful journey through a myriad of poses that not only promote flexibility and strength but also foster creativity, mindfulness, and joy. Let's delve into the intricacies of these poses, exploring their benefits and the imaginative stories that can bring them to life.

1.   Mountain Pose (Tadasana):

Begin the exploration with the foundational Mountain Pose. Standing tall with feet grounded and arms reaching skyward, children embody the strength and stability of a mountain. This pose promotes body awareness, balance, and a sense of groundedness. As children reach for the sky, they are encouraged to visualize themselves as mighty mountains, rooted and unshakable.

2.   Tree Pose (Vrikshasana):

Transitioning into the Tree Pose, children emulate the graceful sway of a tree in the wind. This balancing pose not only enhances physical stability but also encourages focus and concentration. Imagining their bodies as strong, resilient trees, children experience the connection between grounding roots and reaching branches.

3. Downward-Facing Dog (Adho Mukha Svanasana):

Invite children to explore the playful and rejuvenating Downward-Facing Dog pose. Mimicking a curious dog stretching itself, this pose promotes flexibility in the spine and limbs. Children can visualize themselves as friendly dogs, stretching and wagging their imaginary tails, creating a sense of openness and playfulness.

4. Cobra Pose (Bhujangasana):

Transitioning to the Cobra Pose, children embody the grace and strength of a serpent. As they lift their chests off the ground, this backbend encourages flexibility in the spine and opens the heart. Incorporating storytelling, facilitators can guide children to visualize themselves as cobras, exploring the vibrant world around them.

5. Butterfly Pose (Baddha Konasana):

The Butterfly Pose invites children to explore the gentle opening of the hips and the fluttering of butterfly wings. Seated with the soles of their feet together, children can engage in a whimsical exploration of this pose, moving their "butterfly wings" to the rhythm of their breath. This pose encourages flexibility in the hips and a sense of fluidity.

6. Child's Pose (Balasana):

Transitioning to a restful and grounding pose, Child's Pose provides a moment of introspection and relaxation. Children can fold forward, resting their foreheads on the mat with arms stretched out in front. This pose fosters a sense of safety and comfort, encouraging children to take a quiet moment for themselves and reconnect with their breath.

7. Seated Forward Bend (Paschimottanasana):

As children sit with their legs extended forward, the Seated Forward Bend encourages a gentle stretch along the spine and the back of the legs. Incorporating storytelling, facilitators can guide children to visualize reaching for the toes like little explorers, fostering a sense of curiosity and flexibility.

8. Warrior Poses (Virabhadrasana I and II):

Introduce the powerful Warrior Poses, embodying strength and courage. In Warrior I, children reach their arms overhead, imagining themselves as brave warriors facing the sun. Warrior II invites them to stretch their arms in opposite directions, visualizing themselves as warriors gazing into the distance. These poses enhance balance, strength, and a sense of empowerment.

9. Happy Baby Pose (Ananda Balasana):

Transitioning into a playful and delightful pose, the Happy Baby Pose invites children to lie on their backs, holding their feet and rocking gently from side to side. This pose not only promotes hip flexibility but also elicits laughter and a joyful sense of playfulness. Children can envision themselves as happy babies, exploring the world with innocence and delight.

10. Bridge Pose (Setu Bandhasana):

Concluding the exploration of yoga poses with the Bridge Pose, children engage in a gentle backbend that strengthens the legs and opens the chest. Imagining themselves as bridges spanning across a flowing river, children can visualize the support and strength they embody. This pose encourages a sense of stability and resilience.

As children immerse themselves in these yoga poses, the physical benefits intertwine with imaginative storytelling, creating a holistic and engaging experience. Facilitators are encouraged to weave narratives that invite children to visualize themselves as various characters, animals, or elements of nature. This imaginative approach not only enhances the enjoyment of the practice but also deepens the connection between mind and body.

Beyond the physical aspects, these poses become tools for self-expression, creativity, and mindfulness. Children discover the joy of movement and the wonder of their bodies, fostering a positive relationship with physical activity. As facilitators guide them through the playful exploration of yoga poses, they are not only promoting physical health but also laying the foundation for a lifelong journey of self-discovery and well-being. Each pose becomes a stepping stone in the magical world of kids' yoga, where imagination and movement dance hand in hand.

2.1 Gentle Poses for Beginners

Embarking on a yoga journey can be a gentle and nurturing experience, especially for beginners. These poses offer a welcoming introduction to the practice, focusing on ease, relaxation, and the development of foundational skills. Whether you're a newcomer to yoga or guiding beginners, these gentle poses provide a foundation for building flexibility, strength, and a sense of well-being.

1.   **Mountain Pose (Tadasana):**

Begin by standing with feet hip-width apart, grounding through all four corners. Inhale as you reach your arms overhead, palms facing each other. This foundational pose encourages alignment, balance, and a sense of rootedness, setting the stage for the practice.

2.   **Child's Pose (Balasana):**

Transition to Child's Pose for a restful and introspective stretch. Kneel on the mat, sit back on your heels, and extend your arms forward with palms resting on the floor. This pose provides a gentle stretch for the back, hips, and shoulders, fostering a sense of surrender and relaxation.

3.   Downward-Facing Dog (Adho Mukha Svanasana):

Move into Downward-Facing Dog, starting on hands and knees. Lift your hips toward the sky, straighten your legs, and allow your heels to descend toward the mat. This pose offers a gentle stretch for the spine, hamstrings, and calves, while also encouraging full-body engagement.

4.   Cat-Cow Stretch (Marjaryasana-Bitilasana):

From hands and knees, the transition between Cat and Cow poses. Inhale, arch your back, and lift your gaze for Cow Pose. Exhale, round your spine, and tuck your chin for Cat Pose. This gentle flow enhances spinal flexibility and encourages mindful breath with movement.

5.   Seated Forward Bend (Paschimottanasana):

Sit with legs extended in front of you and gently hinge at the hips to reach toward your toes. This seated forward bend provides a gentle stretch for the hamstrings and lower back. Use a soft bend in the knees if needed and focus on reaching forward with a relaxed spine.

6.   Easy Pose (Sukhasana):

Find a comfortable seated position with legs crossed. Rest your hands on your knees, palms facing up or down. Easy Pose is a grounding posture that encourages proper posture, mindful breathing, and a sense of calm.

7. Cobra Pose (Bhujangasana):

Lie on your stomach, place your hands under your shoulders, and lift your chest while keeping your pelvis on the mat. Cobra Pose gently strengthens the back muscles and opens the chest. Ensure the movement is smooth and controlled.

8. Warrior I (Virabhadrasana I):

Step one foot back, keeping the front knee bent over the ankle, and extend your arms overhead. Warrior I is a beginner-friendly standing pose that builds strength in the legs and encourages a gentle opening of the chest.

9. Tree Pose (Vrikshasana):

Stand on one leg, bringing the sole of the other foot to the inner thigh or calf (avoid the knee). Place your hands in a prayer position at your heart or extend them overhead. Tree Pose promotes balance, stability, and a connection to the present moment.

10. Corpse Pose (Savasana):

Conclude the practice with Corpse Pose, lying on your back with legs extended and arms by your sides. Close your eyes and focus on your breath. Savasana allows the body to absorb the benefits of the practice and induces a state of deep relaxation.

Tips for Beginners:

- ***Listen to Your Body***: Pay attention to how your body feels in each pose. Gentle discomfort is normal, but avoid any sharp or painful sensations.
- ***Breathe Mindfully***: Coordinate your breath with movement. Inhale during expansive movements, and exhale during contracting or releasing actions. This mindful breathing enhances the calming aspect of the practice.
- ***Use Props***: Don't hesitate to use props such as blocks, blankets, or straps to support your practice. Props can provide additional stability and make the poses more accessible.
- ***Go at Your Own Pace***: Yoga is a personal journey, and progress is unique to each individual. Honor your body and progress gradually, respecting your current level of flexibility and strength.
- ***Stay Present***: Focus on the present moment and the sensations in your body. Mindful awareness is a fundamental aspect of the yoga practice that promotes relaxation and self-discovery.

As beginners explore these gentle yoga poses, they lay the foundation for a practice that is both accessible and transformative. The emphasis on mindful movement, breath awareness, and self-compassion creates a welcoming space for individuals to nurture their physical and mental well-being.

2.2 Intermediate Poses for Growing Bodies

As young practitioners progress in their yoga journey, intermediate poses provide an opportunity for continued growth, challenge, and exploration. These poses build upon the foundational skills developed in earlier stages and introduce elements that enhance strength, flexibility, and body awareness. Encourage young individuals to explore these intermediate poses with curiosity, mindfulness, and a sense of joy.

1.   **Warrior III (Virabhadrasana III):**

Transition from Warrior I to Warrior III by extending one leg straight back while leaning forward, creating a straight line from the extended heel to the head. This balancing pose strengthens the core, improves focus, and enhances stability in a challenging yet empowering stance.

2.   **Extended Triangle Pose (Utthita Trikonasana):**

From a wide-legged stance, extend one leg out and reach toward the toes on the opposite side. This lateral stretch engages the entire body, promoting flexibility in the spine and legs. Emphasize reaching both up and down simultaneously, creating a long and energized line.

3.   **Chair Pose (Utkatasana):**

Chair Pose is a dynamic pose that strengthens the legs and engages the core. From a standing position, bend the knees and lower the hips as if sitting in an invisible chair. Encourage participants to lift their arms overhead, creating length in the spine while maintaining a strong and active lower body.

4.   Revolved Crescent Lunge (Parivrtta Anjaneyasana):

From a low lunge position, twist the torso towards the bent knee, placing the opposite elbow on the outside of the knee. This revolved variation of Crescent Lunge builds strength in the legs and core while enhancing spinal flexibility. Emphasize the rotation and encourage participants to maintain a steady breath.

5.   Pigeon Pose (Eka Pada Rajakapotasana):

Pigeon Pose is an intermediate hip-opening pose that provides a deep stretch for the hips and thighs. From a tabletop position, bring one knee towards the wrist, extending the other leg straight back. Encourage participants to square their hips and explore the depth of the stretch while maintaining comfort.

6.   Upward-Facing Dog (Urdhva Mukha Svanasana):

Transitioning from Cobra Pose, Upward-Facing Dog involves lifting the chest, straightening the arms, and lifting the thighs off the mat. This backbend strengthens the arms, wrists, and spine while opening the chest. Emphasize the extension of the spine and the engagement of the back muscles.

7.   Side Plank (Vasisthasana):

Side Plank is a challenging yet rewarding pose that builds strength in the core, arms, and wrists. From a plank position, shift weight onto one hand and rotate the body, stacking the feet and lifting the opposite arm towards the sky. Encourage participants to engage the core for stability.

8.   Camel Pose (Ustrasana):

Camel Pose is a backbend that stretches the front of the body while engaging the legs and core. From a kneeling position, reach back to grasp the heels while arching the back. Encourage participants to lift the chest and hips, creating a gentle curve in the spine. Support the neck by keeping it in a neutral position.

9.   Garland Pose (Malasana):

Garland Pose is a deep squat that opens the hips and strengthens the lower body. From a standing position, lower into a squat, bringing the palms together at the heart. Encourage participants to press their elbows against the inner thighs, promoting hip flexibility and stability.

10. Wheel Pose (Urdhva Dhanurasana):

Wheel Pose is an invigorating backbend that strengthens the arms, shoulders, and back while opening the chest. From a supine position, place the hands beside the head, fingers pointing towards the shoulders, and lift the hips towards the sky. Support participants in gradually building up to this pose, emphasizing the importance of proper alignment.

Tips for Practicing Intermediate Poses:

- *Warm-Up Adequately*: Ensure a thorough warm-up to prepare the body for the demands of intermediate poses. Include dynamic movements, gentle stretches, and mindful breathing.
- *Focus on Alignment*: Emphasize proper alignment in each pose to prevent strain and injury. Guide participants to maintain awareness of their body's alignment and make necessary adjustments.
- *Encourage Mindful Breathing*: Remind individuals to maintain a steady and controlled breath throughout the practice. Mindful breathing enhances focus, relaxation, and resilience.
- *Modify as Needed*: Support participants in modifying poses based on their comfort and ability. Provide variations and use props to make the poses accessible and enjoyable.
- *Explore Progress Gradually*: Encourage a gradual and progressive approach to intermediate poses. Celebrate small achievements and acknowledge the evolving strength and flexibility of each participant.

As young bodies grow and develop, intermediate yoga poses offer a pathway to continued physical and mental well-being. The exploration of these poses provides a bridge between foundational movements and more advanced practices, fostering a sense of empowerment and joy in the yoga journey.

2.3 Advanced Yoga Poses for Building Strength and Focus

As practitioners advance in their yoga journey, advanced poses offer a dynamic exploration of strength, flexibility, and heightened mindfulness. These poses challenge the body and mind, requiring a combination of physical prowess, mental focus, and breathe control. Encourage those ready for the next level of their practice to approach these poses with respect, patience, and a sense of curiosity.

1. **Handstand (Adho Mukha Vrksasana):**

Handstand is an invigorating inversion that builds upper body strength, core stability, and balance. Practitioners begin in Downward-Facing Dog, lift one leg, and kick up to bring both legs overhead. Emphasize proper alignment, engage the core, and encourage participants to find stability through the hands and shoulders.

2. **Forearm Stand (Pincha Mayurasana):**

Forearm Stand is a challenging inversion that builds strength in the shoulders, arms, and core. From a Dolphin Pose position, practitioners lift one leg and gradually extend both legs overhead. Support participants in engaging the core, keeping the gaze forward, and finding stability in the forearms.

3.   **Flying Pigeon Pose (Eka Pada Galavasana):**

This arm balance is an advanced variation of Pigeon Pose. In a downward-facing Dog, practitioners bring one knee towards the triceps, lift the back leg, and extend it horizontally. The arms support the body weight, requiring strength in the core and upper body.

4.   **Firefly Pose (Tittibhasana):**

Firefly Pose is an arm balance that challenges strength in the core, arms, and inner thighs. From a squatting position, practitioners place their hands on the mat, hook the knees onto the upper arms, and extend the legs straight forward. Encourage engagement of the core and a gradual lift of the feet off the ground.

5.   **King Pigeon Pose (Kapotasana):**

King Pigeon Pose is a deep backbend that requires flexibility in the spine, shoulders, and quadriceps. From a kneeling position, practitioners reach back to grasp the feet while arching the back. Support participants in gradually easing into the pose, emphasizing proper warm-up and alignment.

6.   **Eight-Angle Pose (Astavakrasana):**

Eight-Angle Pose is an arm balance that combines strength and flexibility. From a seated position, practitioners hook one leg over the arm while extending the other leg. The arms support the body weight as the legs extend, requiring core engagement and balance.

7.   Scorpion Pose (Vrschikasana):

Scorpion Pose is an advanced backbend that challenges the spine's flexibility and strength. From a Forearm Stand position, practitioners slowly lower the legs towards the head, creating a graceful curve. Emphasize controlled movement, engagement of the core, and a strong foundation in the forearms.

8.   Bird of Paradise Pose (Svarga Dvijasana):

Bird of Paradise Pose is a standing pose that combines strength, balance, and hip flexibility. From a standing position, practitioners lift one leg, hook the foot with the hand, and extend the leg to the side. This pose requires a strong foundation in the standing leg and engagement of the core.

9.   Visvamitrasana (Pose Dedicated to the Sage Visvamitra):

Visvamitrasana is a challenging lateral pose that requires strength, flexibility, and balance. From a standing position, practitioners move into a wide-legged stance, reach one arm forward, and lower into a deep lateral stretch. This pose engages the core and promotes a sense of openness in the side body.

10. Lotus Headstand (Padma Sirsasana):

Lotus Headstand combines the meditative aspect of Lotus Pose with the strength and balance of Headstand. Practitioners first come into Lotus Pose, then lift into Headstand with the legs crossed. This advanced inversion requires a strong foundation in the arms, shoulders, and core.

Tips for Practicing Advanced Poses:

- ***Proper Warm-Up***: Ensure a thorough warm-up that includes dynamic movements, targeted stretches, and joint mobility exercises to prepare the body for advanced poses.
- ***Build Strength Gradually***: Progressively build strength through the regular practice of foundational and intermediate poses before attempting advanced poses.
- ***Mindful Alignment***: Emphasize precise alignment to prevent injury and enhance the effectiveness of each pose. Encourage practitioners to stay mindful of their body's position throughout the practice.
- ***Use Props as Needed***: Support practitioners with props such as blocks, straps, or blankets to provide stability and assist in achieving proper alignment in advanced poses.
- ***Focus on Breath Control***: Guide practitioners to maintain steady and controlled breathing. Breath awareness enhances concentration, relaxation, and resilience during challenging poses.
- ***Know Limitations***: Encourage practitioners to listen to their bodies and know their limitations. Advise against pushing beyond a comfortable range of motion to prevent injury.

- ***Seek Guidance***: For those exploring advanced poses, consider seeking guidance from experienced yoga instructors or attending advanced-level classes to receive personalized instruction and corrections.

Advanced yoga poses offer a platform for practitioners to explore the depths of their physical and mental capabilities. As individuals cultivate strength, flexibility, and focus, the advanced practice becomes a transformative journey of self-discovery and empowerment. Approach these poses with a spirit of exploration, patience, and a deep appreciation for the continuous evolution of the yoga practice.

Chapter 3: Breathing Techniques for Young Yogis

In the vibrant world of yoga for young practitioners, the art of breathing takes center stage as a foundational element that intertwines seamlessly with movement, mindfulness, and overall well-being. Chapter 3 invites young yogis and their guides to embark on a journey of breath exploration, introducing them to techniques that cultivate awareness, focus, and a harmonious connection between the body and the breath.

1. Balloon Breath (Dirga Pranayama):

Begin the exploration of breath with the playful Balloon Breath. Instruct young yogis to take a deep inhalation through the nose, expanding their lungs like a balloon filling with air. Then, exhale slowly and completely through pursed lips, visualizing the balloon deflating. This technique encourages full, diaphragmatic breathing, fostering a sense of calm and presence.

2. Bunny Breath (Shitali Pranayama):

Introduce the Bunny Breath, a cooling and calming breath. Instruct young practitioners to curl their tongues or create a small opening between the lips. As they inhale through the tongue or lips, imagine sniffing like a bunny. Exhale gently through the nose. This technique not only promotes breath awareness but also provides a soothing sensation.

3.   Bumblebee Breath (Bhramari Pranayama):

Engage young yogis in the Bumblebee Breath to encourage a tranquil mind. Instruct them to cover their ears with their hands, place their thumbs on the tragus, and take a deep breath in. Upon exhaling, produce a humming sound, mimicking the gentle buzz of a bumblebee. This breath is a delightful way to release tension and promote relaxation.

4.   Star Breath (Sitali Pranayama):

The Star Breath combines breath awareness with mindful movement. Instruct young practitioners to stand with feet hip-width apart. As they inhale, reach their arms overhead, creating a star shape. Upon exhaling, bring the hands to the heart. This dynamic breath technique enhances focus, coordination, and a connection to breath and movement.

5.   Cloud Breath (Nadi Shodhana - Alternate Nostril Breathing):

Guide young yogis through the Cloud Breath, a balancing breath technique. Instruct them to sit comfortably and use the thumb and ring finger to alternately close one nostril while inhaling and exhaling through the other. This breath fosters a sense of balance, clarity, and centeredness.

6. Ocean Breath (Ujjayi Pranayama):

Introduce the soothing Ocean Breath to young practitioners. Instruct them to breathe in and out through the nose, slightly constricting the back of the throat to create a gentle, ocean-like sound. This breath promotes relaxation, deepens breath awareness, and is particularly beneficial during moments of focus and concentration.

7. Dragon Breath (Kapalabhati Pranayama):

The Dragon Breath, also known as Skull Shining Breath, adds an element of playfulness to breathwork. Instruct young yogis to sit comfortably, take a deep inhalation, and exhale forcefully through the nose, engaging the abdominal muscles. This rapid breath energizes the body, clears the mind, and brings a sense of vitality.

8. Candle Breath (Sheetali Pranayama):

Guide young yogis in the Candle Breath, a cooling and calming breath technique. Instruct them to sit comfortably, curl the sides of the tongue, and inhale deeply through the curled tongue. Exhale slowly through the nose. If tongue-curling is challenging, they can mimic the sensation by pursing their lips. This breath helps cool the body and promotes a sense of tranquility.

9.   **Starfish Breath (Anulom Vilom - Nadi Shodhana Variation):**

The Starfish Breath is a variation of Nadi Shodhana that introduces young practitioners to alternate nostril breathing. Instruct them to imagine each finger as a different nostril. As they inhale, close one nostril with the thumb, exhale and switch to the other nostril with the next finger. This playful variation encourages focus, concentration, and breath control.

10.   **Rainbow Breath Visualization:**

Conclude the exploration of breath with the Rainbow Breath Visualization. Instruct young yogis to close their eyes, take slow, deep breaths, and visualize inhaling a spectrum of colors. As they exhale, imagine releasing any stress or tension as a gray cloud. This visualization promotes relaxation, creativity, and a positive connection to the breath.

Tips for Teaching Breathing Techniques to Young Yogis:

- ***Make it Playful***: Infuse a sense of playfulness into breathwork to keep young yogis engaged and curious. Use imagery, storytelling, and creative names for breath techniques.
- ***Encourage Expression***: Allow young practitioners to express how each breath technique makes them feel. Use descriptive language and ask open-ended questions to foster a sense of exploration.
- ***Incorporate Movement***: Combine breathwork with simple movements to enhance the mind-body connection. Movements can

be as simple as reaching, twisting, or swaying to complement the breath.

- *Use Props*: Props like props, visual aids, or soft toys can make breathwork more tangible and enjoyable for young yogis. Consider incorporating props that align with the themes of breath techniques.
- *Create a Safe Environment*: Establish a safe and supportive environment where young yogis feel comfortable exploring their breath. Emphasize the non-competitive nature of breathwork.
- *Be Mindful of Attention Spans*: Keep breathwork sessions brief and dynamic to align with the attention spans of young practitioners. Mix and match techniques to maintain engagement.
- *Integrate into Yoga Sequences*: Seamlessly integrate breathing techniques into yoga sequences. Match breathwork to the theme of the session or specific yoga poses to enhance the overall experience.

As young yogis embark on the journey of breath exploration, they cultivate not only physical well-being but also emotional resilience and mental clarity. Chapter 3 serves as a gateway to a lifelong practice of mindful breathing, empowering young individuals to navigate life's challenges with grace, presence, and a deep connection to their breath.

3.1 The Power of Breath in Kids' Yoga

In the whimsical world of kids' yoga, the breath emerges as a transformative force, weaving its magic through movement, mindfulness, and the boundless imagination of young practitioners. Harnessing the power of breath in kids' yoga goes beyond the rhythmic inhales and exhales—it becomes a gateway to self-discovery, emotional regulation, and a sense of empowered well-being. Let's embark on a journey into the profound impact that conscious breathing holds in the hearts and minds of our little yogis.

1.   Anchoring the Present Moment:

The breath becomes a steadfast anchor, grounding young minds in the present moment. In the whirlwind of youthful energy and ever-changing emotions, the simple act of tuning into the breath provides a moment of stillness. As kids learn to ride the waves of their breath, they cultivate the invaluable skill of being present, fostering awareness and resilience.

2.   Emotional Regulation and Expression:

Breath is a silent storyteller of emotions, and in kids' yoga, it becomes a language for emotional expression and regulation. Guided breathwork empowers young yogis to navigate a spectrum of feelings—from the flutter of excitement to the calming waves of tranquility. By embracing breath as a tool, children learn to express and understand their emotions, fostering emotional intelligence and self-regulation.

3.   Connecting Body and Mind:

The breath serves as a bridge between the physical and the mental realms, connecting the body and mind in a dance of harmony. In the playful exploration of yoga poses, conscious breathing becomes the thread that weaves through each movement. This connection cultivates a holistic understanding of the self, promoting body awareness, coordination, and a sense of unity within.

4.   Enhancing Focus and Concentration:

The rhythmic cadence of breath becomes a gentle guide, leading young minds into a state of focused attention. In the midst of dynamic poses or quiet meditation, conscious breathing acts as a steady companion. By engaging in breath techniques that enhance focus, kids develop a heightened ability to concentrate—a skill that extends beyond the yoga mat into their daily activities and learning experiences.

5.   Fostering Mindfulness and Calm:

Breath is the doorway to mindfulness, inviting young yogis into a realm of calm and tranquility. Mindful breathing exercises, such as the observation of the breath's rise and fall, bring a sense of serenity. Through these practices, children learn to navigate stressors with a mindful pause, cultivating an inner sanctuary of peace that they can access whenever needed.

6.   Building Resilience:

The breath, like a resilient companion, teaches kids the art of adaptation and perseverance. Through intentional breathwork, they discover that even in challenging moments, they hold the power to find balance and ease. This resilience becomes a valuable life skill, empowering them to face the inevitable ups and downs with a sense of inner strength.

7.   Igniting Creativity and Imagination:

The breath becomes the fuel for imaginative exploration in kids' yoga. Creative breath exercises, such as the "Dragon Breath" or "Balloon Breath," transform the act of breathing into a playful adventure. As young minds embrace the power of their breath, they unlock a realm of creativity, where every inhale and exhale carries the potential for exciting stories, journeys, and self-expression.

8.   Cultivating Gratitude and Joy:

Conscious breathing becomes a celebration of life, inviting kids to appreciate the gift of each breath. In moments of gratitude breathwork, they learn to savor the present and acknowledge the beauty around them. This cultivation of gratitude and joy through breath fosters a positive outlook, nurturing a sense of appreciation for the simple pleasures of existence.

9.   Promoting Better Sleep and Relaxation:

The breath becomes a gentle lullaby, guiding young yogis into a realm of relaxation and rest. Bedtime breath routines, like the "Star Breath" or "Candle Breath," become rituals that signal the body and mind to unwind. By incorporating calming breath practices, kids enhance their ability to embrace a restful night's sleep, fostering overall well-being.

10. Empowering Autonomy:

The breath, in its simplicity, becomes a source of personal empowerment for young practitioners. As kids become attuned to their breath, they realize that this innate tool is always within reach. This sense of autonomy over their breath cultivates a foundation of self-efficacy, empowering them to navigate challenges and find a sense of control in various aspects of their lives.

In the heart of kids' yoga, the power of breath unfolds as a dynamic force, touching every aspect of a child's development. Through intentional breath practices, young yogis not only enhance their physical well-being but also embark on a journey of self-discovery, emotional resilience, and joyful exploration. The breath becomes a lifelong companion, guiding them with each inhale and exhale into a world of limitless possibilities, where the magic of the present moment is embraced with open hearts and playful spirits.

3.2 Simple Breathing Exercises for Children

In the enchanting world of children's yoga, introducing simple and engaging breathing exercises can be a delightful way to cultivate mindfulness, focus, and emotional well-being. These exercises are designed to be playful, allowing young minds to connect with their breath in a joyful and imaginative manner. Encourage children to explore these exercises with curiosity and a sense of wonder.

1. **Balloon Breath:**

Instructions:

- Sit comfortably with a straight spine or stand with feet hip-width apart.
- Inhale deeply through the nose, expanding the belly like a balloon.
- Exhale slowly through pursed lips, imagining the balloon deflating.

2. **Bunny Breath:**

Instructions:

- Invite children to sit or stand comfortably.
- Inhale through the nose with short, quick sniffs, imitating a bunny.
- Exhale gently through the nose, maintaining a calm and steady breath.

3. **Star Breath:**

Instructions:

- Stand with feet hip-width apart.
- Inhale as arms reach overhead, creating a star shape.
- Exhale as hands come back to the heart.

- Repeat, coordinating breath with movement.

4.   Dragon Breath:

Instructions:

- Sit comfortably and take a deep breath in.
- Exhale forcefully through the nose, imagining you're breathing out fire like a dragon.
- Repeat several times, embracing the playful intensity.

5.   Candle Breath:

Instructions:

- Sit comfortably with a straight spine.
- Inhale deeply through the nose.
- Exhale slowly through pursed lips, as if blowing out a candle.

6.   Rainbow Breath Visualization:

Instructions:

- Close your eyes and take slow, deep breaths.

- Inhale a spectrum of colors, imagining a rainbow entering with each breath.
- Exhale, releasing any stress or tension as a gray cloud.

7. Ocean Breath:

Instructions:

- Sit comfortably and close your eyes.
- Inhale and exhale through the nose, creating a gentle ocean-like sound by constricting the back of the throat.

8. Butterfly Breath:

Instructions:

- Sit with the soles of the feet together.
- Inhale deeply through the nose.
- Exhale as the wings of the butterfly come together, fluttering softly.

9. Starfish Breath:

Instructions:

- Imagine each finger as a different nostril.
- Inhale through one nostril, switch fingers and exhale through the other nostril.
- Repeat, resembling the arms of a starfish.

10. Scented Flower Breath:

Instructions:

- Encourage children to imagine holding a beautiful scented flower.
- Inhale deeply through the nose, smelling the imaginary flower.
- Exhale slowly through the mouth, as if blowing away the flower's scent.

Tips for Guiding Breathing Exercises:

- ***Create a Playful Atmosphere:***

Infuse a sense of playfulness into the exercises, using creative names, stories, or visualizations to make them engaging.

- ***Keep it Age-Appropriate:***

Tailor the exercises to the age and developmental level of the children, ensuring that they are simple and enjoyable.

- ***Use Props or Imagery:***

Introduce props like scarves or bubbles to make the exercises more visually appealing. Incorporate imagery that resonates with children's imagination.

- ***Encourage Expression:***

Allow children to express how each breathing exercise makes them feel. Use open-ended questions to foster communication.

- ***Incorporate Movement:***

Combine breathwork with simple movements to enhance the mind-body connection. Movements can be as simple as swaying, stretching, or gentle yoga poses.

- ***Be Patient and Supportive:***

Children may take time to embrace these practices. Be patient, and supportive, and encourage a non-judgmental atmosphere.

- ***Make it a Regular Practice:***

Integrate these breathing exercises into a routine, making them a regular part of children's daily activities or as transitions between different tasks.

Breathing exercises for children are not only tools for relaxation but also gateways to developing crucial skills such as mindfulness, emotional awareness, and self-regulation. By infusing these practices with a spirit of playfulness, children can embark on a journey of self-discovery, guided by the magic and joy of their own breath.

3.3 Teaching Mindful Breathing for Stress Relief

In the fast-paced and often hectic landscape of modern life, the practice of mindful breathing stands as a sanctuary, offering individuals a powerful tool for stress relief and relaxation. Whether in a classroom, workplace, or community setting, teaching mindful breathing can empower individuals to navigate stress with resilience and cultivate a sense of inner calm. Here's a guide on how to effectively teach mindful breathing for stress relief:

1. **Create a Comfortable Environment:**

Before diving into the practice, set the stage for a comfortable and safe environment. Ensure that participants have a quiet space to sit or lie down, free from distractions. Consider dimming lights, playing soft background music, or incorporating soothing elements like blankets or cushions.

2.   Explain the Benefits of Mindful Breathing:

Begin by sharing the tangible benefits of mindful breathing. Emphasize that this practice is a scientifically proven method for stress reduction, improved focus, and enhanced overall well-being. Help participants understand that mindful breathing provides a practical and accessible way to respond to stressors in their lives.

3.   Introduce the Basics of Mindful Breathing:

Outline the foundational principles of mindful breathing. Guide participants to focus on the breath as it naturally flows in and out. Emphasize the importance of observing the breath without judgment and with a gentle, curious awareness. Explain that the breath serves as an anchor to the present moment.

4.   Guide a Simple Breathing Exercise:

Lead participants through a simple mindful breathing exercise to experientially understand the practice. One effective exercise is the "4-7-8 Breath":

- Inhale quietly through the nose for a count of 4.
- Hold your breath for a count of 7.
- Exhale audibly through the mouth for a count of 8.
- Encourage participants to repeat this cycle for a few rounds.

5. Cultivate Mindful Awareness:

Guide participants to observe their thoughts, sensations, and emotions without attachment. Remind them that it's normal for the mind to wander, and the key is to gently bring the focus back to the breath. Encourage a non-judgmental attitude toward whatever arises during the practice.

6. Provide Variations for Comfort:

Recognize that individuals have different preferences, and offer variations to suit their comfort. Some may prefer sitting, while others find lying down more relaxing. Allow flexibility in hand placement, whether on the belly, chest, or in a comfortable resting position.

7. Incorporate Mindful Movement:

Integrate gentle movement into the practice for those who find it challenging to stay still. For example, guide participants to mindfully walk in a small area, coordinating each step with their breath. The combination of movement and breath deepens the mind-body connection.

8. Use Guided Imagery and Visualization:

Enhance the mindful breathing experience by incorporating guided imagery or visualization. Encourage participants to envision a serene place, such as a beach or forest, and invite them to engage their senses in this mental sanctuary while continuing to breathe mindfully.

9. Encourage Regular Practice:

Stress the importance of consistency in mindful breathing practice. Recommend incorporating short sessions into daily routines, especially during moments of heightened stress. Consistent practice helps build resilience and reinforces the ability to turn to mindful breathing in times of need.

10. Facilitate Reflection and Discussion:

Conclude the session with a moment for participants to reflect on their experience. Encourage open discussion about how mindful breathing felt for them, any challenges they encountered, and the potential applications in their daily lives. Validate the diverse experiences within the group.

11. Provide Resources for Continued Learning:

Offer resources, such as recommended books, apps, or online guides, to support participants in deepening their understanding of mindful breathing. Providing accessible tools ensures that individuals can continue to explore and integrate mindful breathing into their lives beyond the session.

12. Emphasize Self-Compassion:

Remind participants that mindfulness is a personal journey, and there's no "right" way to practice. Encourage a spirit of self-compassion, where individuals honor their unique experiences and acknowledge that progress comes with patience and continued exploration.

Teaching mindful breathing for stress relief is an invaluable gift, providing individuals with a sustainable and empowering approach to managing the complexities of daily life. By creating a supportive environment, introducing foundational principles, and guiding experiential practices, you empower participants to tap into the transformative potential of their breath, fostering a resilient and grounded approach to stress.

Chapter 4: Incorporating Mindfulness

In the journey of exploring yoga for holistic well-being, the integration of mindfulness becomes a key pillar, enriching the practice with a profound sense of presence, awareness, and connection. This chapter invites practitioners into the art of incorporating mindfulness into their yoga journey, transcending the physical postures to embrace a mindful way of living. Let's delve into the transformative power of weaving mindfulness into every breath, movement, and moment on the mat.

1.   The Essence of Mindfulness in Yoga:

Begin by unraveling the essence of mindfulness in the context of yoga. Delve into the origins of mindfulness practices and their symbiotic relationship with yoga philosophy. Emphasize that mindfulness is not just a technique but a way of being—one that nurtures an awakened presence in each unfolding moment.

2.   Mindful Breath as the Anchor:

Explore the profound connection between mindfulness and the breath. Guide practitioners to understand the breath as a constant anchor, a rhythmic companion that grounds them in the present moment. Offer simple breath awareness exercises to initiate a mindful journey, fostering a deeper connection between breath and consciousness.

3. Embodied Awareness in Asana Practice:

Transition into the physical dimension of yoga by emphasizing embodied awareness during asana practice. Guide practitioners to move with intention, bringing mindful attention to each posture, transition, and nuance of sensation. Encourage a non-judgmental exploration of the body's capabilities and limitations, fostering a compassionate relationship with the self.

4. Mindful Movement and Flow:

Explore the dance of mindful movement, where yoga transitions become a graceful flow of awareness. Introduce flowing sequences that seamlessly integrate breath with movement, allowing practitioners to experience the meditative quality of mindful flow. Emphasize the joy of moving with intention and presence.

5. The Art of Mindful Meditation:

Dive into the art of mindful meditation as a natural extension of the yoga practice. Guide practitioners through mindfulness meditation techniques, such as breath-focused meditation, body scan, or loving-kindness meditation. Illuminate the transformative impact of regular meditation on cultivating inner stillness and a clear, focused mind.

6. Mindful Eating and Yoga Nidra:

Extend mindfulness beyond the mat by exploring mindful eating practices and the restorative realm of Yoga Nidra. Delve into the sensory experience of eating with awareness, savoring each bite as a meditation. Introduce the practice of Yoga Nidra as a guided meditation for profound relaxation, inviting practitioners into a state of conscious rest.

7. Mindfulness in Everyday Life:

Unearth the practical applications of mindfulness in everyday life. Offer insights into incorporating mindfulness into daily routines, such as mindful walking, mindful listening, or mindful breathing breaks. Empower practitioners to carry the essence of mindfulness into their interactions, work, and moments of quiet solitude.

8. Cultivating Gratitude and Mindful Reflection:

Foster the practice of gratitude as a gateway to mindful reflection. Guide practitioners in cultivating gratitude through journaling, reflection, or gratitude walks. Explore how the conscious acknowledgment of blessings and experiences deepens the connection to the present moment.

9. Mindfulness for Emotional Resilience:

Navigate the realm of emotional resilience through mindfulness. Discuss how mindfulness practices can serve as powerful tools for managing stress, anxiety, and emotional challenges. Share techniques for mindfully observing emotions, allowing practitioners to respond with equanimity rather than react impulsively.

10. Mindful Living Beyond the Mat:

Conclude the exploration of mindfulness by emphasizing its integration into daily life. Illuminate how the principles of mindfulness—presence, non-judgment, and awareness—extend beyond the yoga mat. Encourage practitioners to embrace a mindful approach to relationships, work, and self-care, creating a harmonious tapestry of mindful living.

11. Guiding Mindfulness in Yoga Classes:

If applicable, provide guidance for yoga instructors on incorporating mindfulness into their classes. Offer strategies for weaving mindfulness cues into verbal instructions, creating intentional pauses, and fostering a contemplative atmosphere. Emphasize the role of the instructor as a mindful guide.

12. Resources for Further Exploration:

Conclude the chapter by providing resources for further exploration of mindfulness in yoga. Recommend books, podcasts, and online resources that delve into the depths of mindfulness practices, philosophy, and its intersection with yoga.

Incorporating mindfulness into the yoga journey is a profound exploration of the interconnectedness between mind, body, and spirit. This chapter serves as a guide for practitioners to infuse each moment on the mat with mindful awareness, creating a tapestry of presence that extends into the richness of everyday life. As mindfulness becomes a way of living, the transformative power of yoga unfolds, inviting practitioners into a holistic and awakened existence.

4.1 Mindfulness and Its Importance for Kids

In the bustling world of children, where curiosity dances with boundless energy, introducing mindfulness becomes a gift that nurtures emotional well-being, resilience, and a deeper connection to the present moment. Mindfulness, often associated with meditation and contemplation, emerges as a valuable ally in the holistic development of young minds. Let's explore the significance of mindfulness for kids and how it shapes their journey towards a balanced and flourishing life.

1. Fostering Emotional Regulation:

Mindfulness equips children with the tools to navigate the colorful spectrum of emotions. By cultivating awareness of their thoughts and feelings, kids develop the capacity to regulate emotions. Mindfulness practices, such as focused breathing or guided imagery, become anchors that help children respond to situations with calmness and self-assurance.

2. Enhancing Concentration and Focus:

The busy world can be overwhelming for young minds to learn to concentrate. Mindfulness practices, even in short bursts, enhance attention spans and focus. By engaging in activities that require present-moment awareness, kids develop the ability to concentrate on tasks, absorb information more effectively, and approach challenges with a focused mindset.

3. Promoting Stress Reduction:

While the joys of childhood are abundant, so are the occasional stressors. Mindfulness provides a sanctuary—a mental pause button that allows kids to navigate stress with grace. Simple mindfulness exercises, such as deep breathing or mindful coloring, become powerful tools for reducing stress, promoting relaxation, and fostering resilience in the face of challenges.

4. Cultivating Self-Awareness:

Mindfulness invites children into the realm of self-discovery. By encouraging the observation of thoughts, sensations, and emotions without judgment, kids develop a keen sense of self-awareness. This self-awareness becomes a compass, guiding them in understanding their strengths, preferences, and the interconnectedness of their inner world.

5.   Building Healthy Relationships:

The ability to be present and attuned to others is a cornerstone of healthy relationships. Mindfulness practices encourage empathy, active listening, and compassion. As kids learn to be fully present in their interactions, they build strong foundations for meaningful connections with peers, family, and the world around them.

6.   Improving Sleep Quality:

Quality sleep is essential for the growing minds and bodies of children. Mindfulness practices, especially those that focus on relaxation and breath awareness, become valuable tools for improving sleep quality. By cultivating a calm and centered state of mind, kids are better equipped to transition into a restful night's sleep.

7.   Encouraging a Positive Mindset:

Mindfulness fosters a positive mindset by shifting the focus to the present moment. Through practices like gratitude reflection, kids learn to appreciate the positive aspects of their lives. This positive outlook becomes a reservoir of strength, helping children approach challenges with optimism and resilience.

8. Developing Mindful Eating Habits:

The connection between mindfulness and healthy eating habits is profound. Mindful eating practices, such as savoring each bite or paying attention to hunger and fullness cues, instill a sense of mindful nourishment. This awareness fosters a healthy relationship with food and promotes overall well-being.

9. Cultivating a Sense of Calm:

Mindfulness serves as a sanctuary of calm within the whirlwind of childhood activities. By regularly engaging in mindful practices, kids develop an internal refuge—a place of tranquility that they can access during moments of excitement, stress, or overstimulation.

10. Empowering Coping Skills:

Life is filled with ups and downs, and mindfulness equips children with resilient coping skills. By embracing mindfulness, kids learn to respond to challenges with adaptability and creativity. Mindfulness becomes a toolbox of coping strategies that accompany them throughout their lives.

11. Integrating Mindfulness into Education:

Recognizing the profound impact of mindfulness, educators are increasingly integrating it into the classroom. Mindful moments, brief breathing exercises, or mindful transitions between activities contribute to a positive and focused learning environment.

12. Encouraging Playful Mindfulness Practices:

Given the playful nature of childhood, mindfulness can be introduced through enjoyable activities. Mindful games, storytelling, and creative expressions become avenues for weaving mindfulness into the fabric of children's daily lives, making it a natural and enjoyable part of their routine.

In the tapestry of a child's development, mindfulness emerges as a vibrant thread that weaves together emotional intelligence, resilience, and a deep appreciation for the richness of each moment. By introducing mindfulness to kids, we offer them a timeless gift—the ability to navigate the complexities of life with a sense of presence, curiosity, and an open heart.

4.2 Fun Mindfulness Activities for Young Minds

In the lively world of young minds, introducing mindfulness can be an engaging and playful adventure. These fun activities are designed to captivate children's imaginations while fostering mindfulness, helping them discover the joy of being present in the moment. Whether in a classroom, at home, or outdoors, these activities make mindfulness an exciting and accessible experience for young explorers.

1. **Mindful Breathing with Pinwheels:**

Materials:

Pinwheels

Instructions:

- Invite children to sit comfortably with a pinwheel in hand.
- Inhale deeply as they watch the pinwheel spin.
- Exhale slowly, noticing the pinwheel's movement.
- Encourage them to match their breath to the pinwheel's spin, creating a rhythmic and mindful experience.

2. **Nature Scavenger Hunt:**

Materials:

List of nature items (leaves, rocks, flowers, etc.)

Instructions:

- Take children on a nature scavenger hunt, encouraging them to use their senses.
- Invite them to touch, smell, and observe each item mindfully.

- After the hunt, gather to discuss their sensory experiences, promoting awareness of the natural world.

3. Bubble Breaths:

Materials:

Bubbles

Instructions:

- Give each child a small bottle of bubbles.
- Inhale deeply and exhale while blowing bubbles.
- Encourage them to focus on the slow, steady breaths as they create a cascade of bubbles, turning it into a mindful and joyful activity.

4. Yoga Freeze Dance:

Materials:

Music

Instructions:

- Play music and invite children to dance mindfully.
- Pause the music intermittently, prompting them to freeze in a yoga pose.
- Encourage them to breathe and hold the pose, exploring stillness amidst movement.

5.   Mindful Coloring:

Materials:

Coloring sheets and crayons

Instructions:

- Provide intricate coloring sheets and invite children to color mindfully.
- Encourage them to focus on the strokes, colors, and sensations of coloring.
- Afterward, discuss the experience and the emotions that arose during the activity.

6. **Five Senses Exploration:**

Materials:

Various objects with distinct textures, scents, and sounds

Instructions:

- Blindfold each child and present different objects for exploration.
- Encourage them to use their senses to guess the object's features.
- Facilitate a discussion afterward, promoting awareness of sensory experiences.

7. **Mindful Storytelling:**

Materials:

Storybooks

Instructions:

- Choose a story with mindful themes or create one together.
- As you read or tell the story, pause to discuss the characters' feelings, encouraging children to relate them to their own experiences mindfully.

8. **Feather Balancing:**

Materials:

Feathers

Instructions:

- Invite children to balance a feather on their hand or another body part.
- Encourage them to focus on their breath and the gentle movements needed to keep the feather balanced.
- This activity promotes concentration and mindfulness.

9. **Mindful Listening with Bells:**

Materials:

Small bells

Instructions:

- Ring a bell and instruct children to close their eyes and listen mindfully until the sound fades completely.

- Discuss the experience, highlighting the importance of attentive listening.

10. Cloud Watching:

Materials:

Blankets or towels

Instructions:

- Lay on the grass or use blankets to look at the sky.
- Encourage children to observe the clouds mindfully, noting their shapes and movements.
- Share reflections on the peacefulness of cloud-watching.

11. Mindful Tasting:

Materials:

A variety of small snacks

Instructions:

- Present different snacks for a mindful tasting experience.
- Encourage children to explore the colors, textures, and flavors of each snack.
- Discuss their observations and preferences.

12. Gratitude Jar:

Materials:

Jar and slips of paper

Instructions:

- Provide each child with a jar and slips of paper.
- Ask them to write one thing they are grateful for each day and place it in the jar.
- Regularly reflect on the collected notes, fostering a culture of gratitude.

These fun mindfulness activities for young minds transform the practice of mindfulness into an exciting journey of self-discovery and present-moment awareness. Through play and exploration, children can develop valuable skills for emotional well-being, focus, and a lifelong appreciation for the richness of each moment.

4.3 Fostering Emotional Well-being through Mindful Practices

In the tapestry of our lives, emotions are vibrant threads that weave through our experiences. Fostering emotional well-being involves cultivating a mindful relationship with these emotions, acknowledging them with compassion, and navigating their currents with grace. This chapter explores the profound impact of incorporating mindful practices into daily life as a pathway to emotional resilience, self-awareness, and a deeper connection to the richness of our emotional landscape.

1. **Understanding the Mind-Emotion Connection:**

Begin by unraveling the intricate connection between the mind and emotions. Explore how thoughts influence emotions and, conversely, how emotions shape our mental landscape. Introduce the concept of mindfulness as a tool for observing and understanding the interplay between thoughts and emotions.

2. **Cultivating Emotional Awareness:**

Dive into the heart of mindfulness by emphasizing the cultivation of emotional awareness. Guide individuals in becoming keen observers of their emotional states without judgment. Encourage the practice of identifying, labeling, and exploring the nuances of emotions, fostering a deep sense of self-awareness.

3.   Mindful Breathing for Emotional Regulation:

Explore the transformative power of mindful breathing as a cornerstone for emotional regulation. Introduce simple breath awareness exercises that individuals can turn to in moments of heightened emotions. Emphasize the role of the breath as a calming anchor that provides a sanctuary amidst the storms of emotions.

4.   Mindful Body Scan for Emotional Release:

Guide individuals through a mindful body scan, inviting them to explore how emotions manifest in the body. This practice encourages the release of physical tension associated with emotions and enhances the mind-body connection. Participants learn to observe sensations without attachment, fostering a sense of ease.

5.   Loving-Kindness Meditation for Emotional Resilience:

Introduce loving-kindness meditation as a powerful tool for cultivating emotional resilience and compassion. Guide individuals to extend heartfelt wishes of well-being to themselves and others. This practice fosters a positive emotional outlook and strengthens the capacity to respond to challenges with kindness.

6.   Mindful Journaling for Emotional Reflection:

Explore the therapeutic benefits of mindful journaling. Encourage individuals to express their emotions through writing, fostering a reflective space for emotional exploration. Provide prompts that guide them in examining the roots of emotions and discovering patterns in their emotional landscape.

7.   Mindful Walking for Emotional Grounding:

Integrate mindfulness into movement with mindful walking practices. Guide individuals to synchronize their steps with their breath, creating a moving meditation. This practice promotes a sense of groundedness, allowing individuals to bring mindful awareness to each step and, by extension, to each moment.

8.   Mindful Listening for Emotional Connection:

Emphasize the role of mindful listening in nurturing emotional connections with others. Explore how attentive listening without judgment fosters empathy and strengthens relationships. Introduce mindful communication practices that encourage individuals to express themselves authentically and with awareness.

9.   Mindful Pause for Emotional Response:

Explore the concept of the mindful pause—a brief moment of stillness before responding to emotions or external stimuli. Guide individuals to use this pause to check in with their emotional state and choose intentional responses. This practice empowers them to navigate situations with mindfulness rather than react impulsively.

10. Mindful Eating for Emotional Nourishment:

Examine the connection between mindful eating and emotional nourishment. Guide individuals to savor each bite with full awareness, fostering a healthy relationship with food. Explore how mindful eating can address emotional eating patterns and promote a sense of satisfaction and well-being.

11. Mindful Art and Creativity for Emotional Expression:

Tap into the expressive power of art and creativity as a means of emotional expression. Encourage individuals to engage in mindful art activities that allow emotions to unfold on canvas or paper. Explore the liberating and therapeutic nature of creative expression in the context of emotional well-being.

12. Mindful Reflection and Gratitude:

Conclude the chapter with practices that emphasize mindful reflection and gratitude. Guide individuals to reflect on their emotional journeys, acknowledging growth and resilience. Explore gratitude practices that cultivate an appreciation for the spectrum of emotions, fostering a positive and balanced emotional landscape.

13. Integrating Mindful Practices into Daily Life:

Empower individuals to integrate mindful practices seamlessly into their daily routines. Discuss the importance of consistency and offer practical tips for incorporating mindfulness into activities such as commuting, household chores, or work responsibilities. Highlight the cumulative impact of small, mindful moments.

14. Resources for Ongoing Emotional Well-being:

Conclude the chapter by providing resources for continued exploration of mindful practices and emotional well-being. Recommend books, apps, or online platforms that support individuals in deepening their understanding and commitment to emotional health.

In the journey of fostering emotional well-being through mindful practices, individuals embark on a transformative exploration of their inner landscape. Mindfulness becomes a guiding light, illuminating the intricate tapestry of emotions with clarity, compassion, and an unwavering presence. Through these practices, individuals cultivate the skills to navigate the ever-changing currents of emotions with resilience, authenticity, and a deep sense of well-being.

Chapter 5: Making Yoga Fun

Yoga is not just a series of poses; it's a playful exploration of mind, body, and spirit. In this chapter, we dive into the art of making yoga a joyous and engaging experience for all ages. Whether you're a yoga instructor, parent, or enthusiast, discover creative approaches to infuse laughter, curiosity, and excitement into every yoga session. Let's explore the realm of making yoga an irresistibly fun adventure.

1. Embarking on a Yoga Adventure:

Begin by framing yoga as a thrilling adventure. Create imaginative narratives that transport participants to magical realms, inviting them to embody different characters or animals through yoga poses. This approach sparks enthusiasm and taps into the innate playfulness of yoga.

2. Yoga Games for All Ages:

Introduce a repertoire of yoga games that transform the mat into a playground. From yoga dice that determine poses to yoga card games that encourage teamwork, infuse the session with the spirit of play. Games not only make yoga enjoyable but also enhance coordination, balance, and social interaction.

3. Music and Movement Fusion:

Elevate the energy of the yoga session by incorporating music and movement. Create themed playlists that match the mood of the practice—whether it's a jungle adventure or an ocean escapade. Encourage participants to express themselves through dance, incorporating yoga poses seamlessly into the rhythmic flow.

4.   Storytime Yoga:

Merge storytelling with yoga by weaving narratives that unfold through poses. Whether it's a classic fable, a nature-inspired tale, or an original adventure, stories make yoga relatable and captivating. Participants embody characters and actions, making the practice an immersive and entertaining experience.

5.   Yoga Art and Creativity:

Tap into the artistic side of yoga by incorporating creative expression. Introduce activities such as mindful coloring of yoga-themed pages, crafting DIY yoga props, or even designing personalized yoga mats. This artistic integration adds a layer of enjoyment to the practice while fostering self-expression.

6.   Yoga Challenges and Achievements:

Make yoga a thrilling journey of achievements by setting challenges. Whether it's holding a pose for an extended time, mastering a new sequence, or creating playful yoga duets, challenges add an element of friendly competition and accomplishment to the practice.

7.   Yoga for Imaginary Play:

Encourage the use of imagination by incorporating props and visuals. From magical wands for balancing poses to imaginary surfboards for standing poses, props make yoga an imaginative playground. This approach not only enhances engagement but also nurtures creativity.

8.   Animal-Inspired Yoga:

Transform the mat into a zoo or safari with animal-inspired yoga. Each pose represents a different creature, allowing participants to embody the spirit of various animals. This not only adds an element of fun but also fosters an appreciation for the diversity of movement in the animal kingdom.

9.   Partner and Group Poses:

Explore the dynamics of connection by introducing partner and group poses. From tree pose partnerships to creating human mandalas, cooperative poses enhance camaraderie and communication. This social aspect transforms yoga into a shared adventure, making it doubly enjoyable.

10. Yoga through Playful Props:

Elevate the fun factor with the addition of playful props. Incorporate items like hula hoops, scarves, or balloons to create dynamic and interactive sequences. Props add an element of surprise, transforming traditional poses into exciting, new adventures.

11. Seasonal and Holiday-Themed Yoga:

Celebrate the changing seasons and holidays by infusing yoga with thematic elements. Whether it's Halloween-inspired poses, winter wonderland sequences, or spring-themed flows, aligning yoga with the rhythm of the seasons makes the practice timely, relevant, and festive.

12. Yoga as a Mindful Celebration:

Conclude each yoga session with a mindful celebration. Create a ritual that marks the end of the practice, such as a gratitude circle, a collective breath, or a simple mindfulness moment. This brings closure to the session on a positive and reflective note.

13. Inclusive and Adaptive Yoga:

Ensure that the fun of yoga is accessible to everyone by embracing inclusivity and adaptability. Provide modifications for poses, encourage creativity in movement, and celebrate the uniqueness of each participant. This approach fosters a supportive and joyful yoga community.

14. Encouraging Laughter Yoga:

Embrace the therapeutic power of laughter yoga. Introduce laughter exercises and playful activities that promote genuine laughter. Laughter not only releases endorphins but also creates a joyful and light-hearted atmosphere, transforming the yoga session into a laughter-filled celebration.

15. Feedback and Reflection:

Conclude the chapter by seeking feedback from participants and reflecting on the fun elements that resonated most. Embrace an iterative approach, incorporating new ideas and adapting the fun elements based on the preferences and experiences of the participants.

Embark on the journey of making yoga an exhilarating and joyous adventure. By infusing creativity, playfulness, and inclusivity into each session, you transform the yoga mat into a magical space where laughter, exploration, and well-being seamlessly converge. The chapter on making yoga fun is an invitation to celebrate the boundless joy that arises when yoga becomes not just a practice but a delightful and transformative experience for all.

5.1 Creative Games and Activities for Kids' Yoga

Engaging children in yoga involves tapping into their natural curiosity and boundless energy. The fusion of playfulness and yoga creates a dynamic and enjoyable experience that nurtures both physical well-being and mindfulness. This chapter introduces a collection of creative games and activities designed to make kids' yoga sessions not just beneficial but downright fun. Let's embark on this playful journey of movement, imagination, and laughter.

1.   Yoga Freeze Dance:

Objective:

Combine music and movement to enhance flexibility and coordination.

Instructions:

- Play music and encourage children to dance freely.
- Pause the music intermittently, prompting them to freeze in a yoga pose.
- Resume dancing when the music restarts.

2.   Yoga Obstacle Course:

Objective:

Develop agility, balance, and focus.

Instructions:

- Set up a course with yoga mats, cones, and other props.
- Designate yoga poses at different stations.
- Children navigate the course, striking a pose at each station.

3. Musical Mats:

Objective:

Enhance listening skills and coordination.

Instructions:

- Arrange yoga mats in a circle, one fewer than the number of participants.
- Play music as children walk or hop around the mats.
- When the music stops, they must quickly find a mat to stand on.

4. Yoga Simon Says:

Objective:

Foster focus and body awareness.

Instructions:

- Take turns being "Simon" and guide children to perform yoga poses.
- Only perform poses when preceded by "Simon says."

5. Animal Yoga Adventure:

Objective:

Introduce yoga poses through imaginative play.

Instructions:

- Assign each child an animal and guide them to mimic the animal's movements.
- Incorporate corresponding yoga poses for each animal.

6. Yoga Storytelling:

Objective:

Combine storytelling with yoga to enhance creativity.

Instructions:

- Tell a story that includes yoga poses.
- Children act out the poses as the story unfolds.

7. Pass the Yoga Pose:

Objective:

Encourage teamwork and cooperation.

Instructions:

- Have children sit in a circle and pass a beanbag or soft object.
- Each child names a yoga pose before passing the object.

8. Yoga Dice Challenge:

Objective:

Introduce variety and excitement to yoga poses.

Instructions:

- Create dice with different yoga poses on each side.
- Children take turns rolling the dice and performing the indicated pose.

9. Yoga Alphabet Hunt:

Objective:

Combine literacy and movement through yoga.

Instructions:

- Scatter alphabet cards around the space.
- As children find each letter, they perform a yoga pose starting with that letter.

10. Yoga Memory Game:

Objective:

Enhance memory and concentration through yoga poses.

- Create pairs of cards with pictures of yoga poses.
- Children take turns flipping over cards to find matching poses.

11. Rainbow Yoga:

Objective:

Explore a variety of poses with color coordination.

Instructions:

- Assign a color to each yoga pose.
- Call out colors, and children perform the corresponding pose.

12. Yoga Sculptures:

Objective:

Promote creativity and collaboration.

Instructions:

- Divide children into small groups.
- Each group creates a "yoga sculpture" by combining their bodies into a pose.

13. Weather Yoga:

Objective:

Connect yoga poses with different weather conditions.

Instructions:

- Call out weather conditions, and children perform poses that reflect each weather type.

14. Yoga Charades:

Objective:

Enhance creativity and body awareness.

Instructions:

- Write various yoga poses on cards.
- Children take turns acting out the poses while others guess.

15. Partner Poses and Mirroring:

Objective:

Foster cooperation and connection.

Instructions:

- Pair children and guide them through partner yoga poses.
- Encourage mirroring, with one child leading and the other following.

These creative games and activities infuse the world of yoga with laughter, imagination, and exploration. By combining movement with playfulness, children not only reap the physical benefits of yoga but also develop essential life skills such as teamwork, concentration, and creativity. This chapter is an invitation to create a vibrant and enjoyable space where kids can flourish on their yoga journey.

5.2 Music and Movement: Enhancing the Joy of Yoga

In the world of yoga, the union of breath, movement, and mindfulness creates a harmonious symphony. Introducing music to this symphony adds a dynamic layer, infusing energy, rhythm, and joy into the practice. This chapter explores the transformative power of music and movement in the realm of yoga, turning the mat into a vibrant stage where each breath is a note and every poses a dance. Join the rhythm of this exploration as we uncover the ways in which music enhances the joy of yoga.

1. The Dance of Breath and Beat:

Begin by recognizing the inherent connection between breath and beat. Music serves as the heartbeat of the yoga practice, guiding the rhythm of breath and movement. Explore the nuances of synchronizing breath with music, creating a dance that invites practitioners into a deeper state of flow and presence.

2. Creating Yoga Playlists:

Delve into the art of crafting yoga playlists that resonate with the theme and energy of the practice. From calming melodies for gentle flows to upbeat tunes for dynamic sequences, the playlist becomes a soundtrack that elevates the emotional and physical experience of yoga. Share insights on selecting music that complements the intention of each session.

3. Rhythmic Flow of Asanas:

Explore the integration of music into the flow of asanas. Guide practitioners through sequences where poses seamlessly align with the musical cadence. Emphasize the joy of moving in harmony with the rhythm, encouraging fluid transitions that transform the practice into a graceful dance.

4. Live Music Experiences:

Uncover the transformative impact of live music in yoga sessions. Whether through live musicians or carefully curated live recordings, the vibrancy and spontaneity of live music elevate the energy of the space. Discuss the ways in which live music fosters a unique and immersive yoga experience.

5. Chants, Mantras, and Sonic Meditation:

Introduce the power of chants, mantras, and sonic meditation as integral elements of the yoga practice. Explore how sacred sounds and vocalizations complement traditional poses, fostering a sense of sacred resonance. Guide practitioners in incorporating chanting into their personal practice for a holistic mind-body experience.

6. Dance-Inspired Yoga Sequences:

Infuse the spirit of dance into yoga sequences. Explore movement-inspired sequences that draw inspiration from various dance forms, encouraging practitioners to express themselves through fluid and expressive postures. Highlight the joyful connection between dance, music, and yoga.

7.   Musical Breath Awareness:

Dive into the practice of musical breath awareness, where the rhythm of the breath aligns with specific beats or melodies. Guide practitioners to use music as a focal point for breath awareness, creating a rhythmic meditation that enhances mindfulness and presence.

8.   Musical Meditation and Savasana:

Explore the use of music in meditation and Savasana. Introduce soothing melodies or ambient sounds that support a deep state of relaxation. Discuss the art of selecting music that nurtures a tranquil and meditative atmosphere, allowing practitioners to surrender into the stillness of Savasana.

9.   Incorporating Cultural Sounds:

Celebrate the richness of cultural diversity through the incorporation of diverse musical genres and sounds. From traditional instruments to contemporary beats, explore how cultural elements in music can deepen the global tapestry of yoga. Encourage practitioners to embrace the global influences that resonate with their practice.

10. Music for Kids' Yoga Adventures:

Adapt the use of music for kids' yoga, transforming the mat into a playful adventure. Explore upbeat and imaginative tunes that accompany themed yoga journeys for children. Discuss how music enhances engagement and encourages creativity in the younger yoga enthusiasts.

11. Mindful Listening and Soundscapes:

Emphasize the practice of mindful listening and the use of soundscapes in yoga. Guide practitioners to attune their awareness to the sounds around them, creating a mindful backdrop that enriches the yoga experience. Discuss the integration of nature sounds, gentle instruments, or ambient recordings for a sensory-rich practice.

12. Dance Party Yoga:

Celebrate the joyous fusion of dance and yoga with a dance party yoga session. Create a vibrant atmosphere where practitioners move freely to uplifting tunes, seamlessly transitioning between dance and yoga poses. Emphasize the liberating and joyful nature of this dynamic practice.

13. Music as an Emotional Catalyst:

Explore the emotional impact of music in yoga. Discuss how specific genres, rhythms, or melodies can evoke different emotions and enhance the emotional release within the practice. Guide practitioners to embrace the emotional journey facilitated by the synergy of music and movement.

14. Yoga Festivals and Musical Collaborations:

Delve into the world of yoga festivals and collaborative experiences with musicians. Discuss the magic that unfolds when yoga and music come together in large gatherings. Share insights on how such events foster community, celebration, and a shared sense of joy.

15. Creating Personal Soundtracks for Home Practice:

Conclude the chapter by empowering practitioners to curate personal soundtracks for their home practice. Encourage them to explore their musical preferences and create playlists that resonate with their unique journey on the mat. Emphasize the role of music as a supportive companion in their individual yoga adventures.

In the realm of yoga, where movement is a language and breath is a melody, the addition of music transforms the practice into a symphony of joy. This chapter is an invitation to explore the harmonious dance of breath and beat, the expressive flow of asanas, and the transformative power of music and movement. By embracing the union of yoga and music, practitioners embark on a dynamic and joyful journey where every pose becomes a note, and every breath, a melody.

6.3 Partner and Group Yoga for Social Connection

Yoga is often viewed as a personal journey, an individual exploration of mind and body. However, the practice also holds the power to foster profound connections between individuals. In this chapter, we delve into the world of partner and group yoga—a dimension where the joy of movement is shared, and the bonds of community are strengthened. Join the exploration of practices that transcend the solitary mat, embracing the spirit of togetherness, communication, and social connection.

1.   The Essence of Partner and Group Yoga:

Begin by illuminating the essence of partner and group yoga. Explore how shared movement enhances communication, trust, and the sense of interconnectedness. Discuss the unique benefits of practicing yoga in pairs or groups, including increased motivation, encouragement, and the joy of collective energy.

2.   Building Trust through Partner Yoga:

Delve into the practice of partner yoga as a means to build trust and connection. Guide participants through partner poses that require mutual support and cooperation. Emphasize the role of trust in enhancing the depth of the practice and creating a safe space for vulnerability and exploration.

3.   Communication and Connection in Pairs:

Explore how partner yoga serves as a platform for communication and connection. Discuss the importance of clear verbal and non-verbal communication during partner poses. Guide participants to develop sensitivity and responsiveness to their partner's movements, fostering a deeper understanding and connection.

4.   Group Dynamics in Yoga:

Uncover the dynamics of practicing yoga in larger groups. Discuss how group yoga sessions create a collective energy that transcends individual practice. Explore the sense of unity and shared intention that arises in a group setting, enhancing the overall experience of the practice.

5.   Encouraging Inclusivity in Group Yoga:

Emphasize the importance of inclusivity in group yoga settings. Discuss strategies for ensuring that everyone feels welcome and supported, regardless of experience or ability. Guide participants to embrace the diversity within the group, fostering an inclusive and supportive yoga community.

6.   Partner Poses for All Levels:

Explore a repertoire of partner poses suitable for practitioners of all levels. From foundational poses that build trust to more advanced poses that challenge balance and coordination, guide participants through a spectrum of partner poses. Highlight modifications to accommodate varying skill levels within pairs.

7.   Partner Yoga Sequences:

Share partner yoga sequences that encourage a fluid and connected practice. Guide participants through sequences that seamlessly transition between partner poses, creating a dynamic flow. Discuss the benefits of moving together, breathing in unison, and cultivating a shared rhythm.

8. Group Yoga Challenges:

Introduce challenges and activities that enhance the sense of connection within a group. From synchronized poses to group balances, encourage participants to explore their collective potential. Discuss the role of challenges in fostering teamwork, communication, and a shared sense of accomplishment.

9. Partner Breathing Exercises:

Explore the intimate connection of breath through partner breathing exercises. Guide participants in synchronized breathing, mirroring each other's inhalations and exhalations. Discuss how shared breath enhances the sense of unity and presence in the practice.

10. Laughing Yoga in Groups:

Embrace the element of joy in group yoga with laughter yoga exercises. Introduce playful activities that encourage genuine laughter within the group. Discuss the therapeutic benefits of laughter, including stress reduction, increased endorphin levels, and the creation of a lighthearted and joyful atmosphere.

11. Mindful Group Meditations:

Transition into the realm of mindfulness with group meditation practices. Guide participants through mindful breathing and visualization exercises that promote a collective sense of calm and presence. Discuss the power of shared stillness in creating a harmonious group energy.

12. Couples Yoga for Connection:

Extend the exploration to couples yoga, emphasizing the connection between romantic partners. Discuss how couples yoga can deepen the emotional bond, enhance communication, and foster a sense of intimacy. Guide couples through poses that encourage mutual support and shared movement.

13. Creating Yoga Circles:

Explore the symbolism and energy of yoga circles. Discuss how forming a circle enhances the sense of equality and interconnectedness within a group. Guide participants through poses and activities that leverage the circular arrangement, creating a supportive and inclusive space.

14. Themed Group Yoga Sessions:

Infuse creativity into group yoga sessions with themed practices. From nature-inspired themes to celebratory occasions, guide participants through practices that resonate with a collective intention. Discuss the role of themes in enhancing group cohesion and creating memorable shared experiences.

15. Community-Building Yoga Events:

Conclude the chapter by exploring community-building yoga events. Discuss the organization of group yoga sessions in community settings, such as parks, schools, or workplaces. Share insights on how these events foster a sense of belonging, build social connections, and contribute to the well-being of the larger community.

In the realm of partner and group yoga, the mat becomes a canvas for shared movement, laughter, and connection. This chapter invites participants to explore the transformative power of practicing yoga together, cultivating a sense of community that extends beyond the individual mat. Through the joy of shared movement, communication, and mutual support, partner and group yoga become gateways to a deeper understanding of ourselves and others.

Chapter 6: Yoga for Different Age Groups

Yoga is a timeless practice that transcends age, embracing individuals at every stage of life. In this chapter, we explore the nuanced approach to yoga tailored for various age groups. From the playful energy of children to the transformative practices for adults and the gentle adaptations for seniors, each age group brings its own unique characteristics and considerations to the mat. Join us in navigating the diverse landscape of age-appropriate yoga, honoring the individual needs, aspirations, and potentials of practitioners at every age.

1. **Yoga for Children:**

Introduction:

- Dive into the world of children's yoga, where imagination, playfulness, and creativity intertwine.

Key Considerations:

Explore the importance of making yoga fun, incorporating storytelling, and adapting poses to cater to the developmental stages of children.

Activities and Games:

Introduce creative games, themed yoga adventures, and activities that engage children's natural curiosity and enthusiasm.

Mindfulness for Kids:

Discuss age-appropriate mindfulness practices to nurture emotional intelligence and self-awareness in children.

2. Yoga for Teens and Adolescents:

Introduction:

Navigate the dynamic landscape of yoga for teens, acknowledging the physical, emotional, and social transformations during adolescence.

Empowering Practices:

Discuss how yoga can empower teens by enhancing self-esteem, promoting body positivity, and providing tools for stress management.

Mind-Body Connection:

Explore practices that foster a strong mind-body connection, helping teens navigate the challenges of self-discovery and identity formation.

Group Dynamics:

Introduce group activities and partner yoga to encourage positive social interactions and a sense of community among adolescents.

3. Yoga for Adults:

Introduction:

Uncover the multifaceted benefits of yoga for adults, addressing physical fitness, mental well-being, and stress reduction.

Holistic Wellness:

Discuss the role of yoga in promoting holistic wellness, including improved flexibility, strength, balance, and enhanced mental clarity.

Adapting to Individual Needs:

Recognize the diversity of adult practitioners and explore how yoga can be adapted to accommodate different fitness levels, health conditions, and lifestyles.

Mindful Living:

Highlight the integration of yoga philosophy into daily life, fostering mindfulness, gratitude, and a balanced approach to challenges.

4.   Prenatal and Postnatal Yoga:

Introduction:

Explore the transformative journey of motherhood and the role of yoga in supporting women during prenatal and postnatal stages.

Prenatal Practices:

Discuss safe and gentle yoga practices for expectant mothers, emphasizing breath awareness, pelvic floor exercises, and relaxation techniques.

Postnatal Recovery:

Address postnatal yoga practices that aid in physical recovery, strengthen the core, and provide nurturing self-care for new mothers.

Bonding with Baby:

Introduce practices that facilitate bonding between mothers and infants, including baby yoga and mindful interactions.

5. Yoga for Midlife and Beyond:

Introduction:

Navigate the evolving landscape of yoga for individuals in midlife and beyond, emphasizing the role of yoga in promoting healthy aging.

Functional Movement:

Explore yoga practices that focus on functional movement, joint flexibility, and balance to support the changing needs of the body.

Mindfulness for Seniors:

Discuss the integration of mindfulness and meditation practices to enhance cognitive function, emotional well-being, and overall quality of life for seniors.

Community Connection:

Highlight the importance of creating inclusive and supportive yoga communities for seniors, fostering social connections and a sense of belonging.

6.   Yoga for Special Populations:

Introduction:

Acknowledge the diverse needs of special populations, including individuals with disabilities, chronic illnesses, or specific health conditions.

Adaptations and Modifications:

Explore how yoga can be adapted to accommodate various abilities and conditions, emphasizing inclusivity and accessibility.

Therapeutic Benefits:

Discuss the therapeutic benefits of yoga for specific populations, including pain management, stress reduction, and improved overall well-being.

Community Support:

Advocate for the creation of supportive and compassionate yoga communities that cater to the unique needs of special populations.

7.   Intergenerational Yoga:

Introduction:

Embrace the concept of intergenerational yoga, fostering connections between different age groups within families or communities.

Shared Practices:

Discuss how shared yoga practices can strengthen familial bonds, promote mutual understanding, and create a sense of unity.

Building Bridges:

Explore the potential for intergenerational yoga to bridge generational gaps, facilitating communication and shared experiences among family members.

Creating Inclusive Spaces:

Advocate for the creation of inclusive yoga spaces that welcome practitioners of all ages, encouraging intergenerational participation and collaboration.

8.   Adapting Yoga for Various Environments:

Introduction:

Recognize the diverse environments in which yoga can be practiced, from schools and workplaces to community centers and healthcare settings.

Educational Settings:

Discuss the integration of yoga into educational settings, emphasizing its benefits for students' focus, emotional regulation, and overall well-being.

Corporate Wellness:

Explore the role of yoga in corporate wellness programs, addressing stress management, employee engagement, and a healthy work-life balance.

Healthcare and Rehabilitation:

Highlight the therapeutic applications of yoga in healthcare and rehabilitation settings, supporting individuals in their journey toward physical and mental recovery.

9. Cultural Considerations in Age-Appropriate Yoga:

Introduction:

Acknowledge the cultural diversity within the practice of yoga and explore how cultural considerations influence age-appropriate yoga approaches.

Cultural Sensitivity:

Discuss the importance of cultural sensitivity in yoga instruction, respecting diverse backgrounds, traditions, and belief systems.

Incorporating Cultural Elements:

Explore ways to incorporate cultural elements, music, and traditions into age-appropriate yoga practices, creating a rich and inclusive experience for practitioners.

10. Resources for Age-Appropriate Yoga:

Introduction:

Provide a comprehensive list of resources, including books, online platforms, and organizations, to support instructors, practitioners, and caregivers in exploring age-appropriate yoga.

Training and Certification:

Highlight the importance of specialized training and certification for instructors working with specific age groups or special populations.

Community Engagement:

- Encourage community engagement and networking, fostering collaboration among yoga professionals, healthcare practitioners, educators, and individuals interested in age-appropriate yoga.

Reflective Integration:

Summarize the diverse approaches explored in age-appropriate yoga, emphasizing the adaptability and inclusivity of the practice across the lifespan.

Invitation to Exploration:

Encourage readers to continue exploring and tailoring yoga practices for various age groups, recognizing the transformative potential of yoga in fostering well-being at every stage of life.

This chapter serves as a guide to the multifaceted world of age-appropriate yoga, celebrating the diversity of practitioners and the adaptability of yoga across the lifespan. Whether introducing children to the joy of movement, empowering adolescents, supporting adults in their wellness journey, or fostering healthy aging, the practice of yoga becomes a lifelong companion, adapting to the evolving needs of individuals and communities.

6.1 Tailoring Practices for Toddlers

Embarking on the journey of introducing yoga to toddlers requires a delightful blend of creativity, patience, and a deep understanding of the boundless energy and curiosity inherent in these little ones. In this section, we'll explore how to tailor yoga practices specifically for toddlers, creating an environment that fosters both physical development and a sense of joyous exploration.

1. **Introduction to Toddler Yoga:**

Understanding Toddler Development:

Recognize the unique physical and cognitive development stages toddlers undergo, shaping their abilities and interests.

Importance of Playfulness:

Embrace the spirit of playfulness as a cornerstone of toddler yoga, acknowledging that learning occurs through joyful exploration.

2. Setting the Stage:

Safe and Inviting Space:

Create a safe and inviting space that encourages toddlers to explore movement freely. Clear any potential hazards and use colorful mats or props to capture their attention.

Use of Props:

Introduce simple and age-appropriate props like soft toys, scarves, or colorful balls to make the practice engaging and interactive.

3. Breathing Activities for Toddlers:

Gentle Breathing Awareness:

Introduce basic breathing awareness through playful activities. Use bubbles and encourage toddlers to take slow breaths, associating the release of bubbles with gentle exhalations.

Imaginative Breathing:

Incorporate imaginative elements into breathing exercises, such as pretending to blow up balloons or being a "birthday candle" that flickers with each breath.

4. Simple Yoga Poses for Toddlers:

Animal-Inspired Poses:

Engage toddlers by introducing animal-inspired poses. Explore gentle and familiar poses like "Downward Dog" (stretching like a dog) or "Cat-Cow" (arching and rounding the back).

Nature-Inspired Poses:

Connect yoga to nature by incorporating poses inspired by elements like trees, flowers, or the sun. Keep the language simple and use visual cues to guide their movements.

5. Storytelling through Movement:

Narrative Yoga Adventures:

Weave simple narratives into the yoga practice, creating short stories that involve movement and imagination. For example, embark on a journey to the jungle, encouraging poses like "Elephant Stomp" or "Butterfly Flutter."

Interactive Storytime Yoga:

Integrate storytelling and movement by inviting toddlers to act out parts of a story. Use props or simple costumes to enhance the imaginative experience.

6. **Music and Rhythm in Toddler Yoga:**

Upbeat and Playful Music:

Choose lively and age-appropriate music to infuse energy into the practice. Use musical cues to transition between poses or activities.

Rhythmic Movement Games:

Incorporate rhythmic movement games that sync with the music. Encourage toddlers to clap, stomp, or sway in tune with the rhythm.

7. **Partner Poses with Caregivers:**

Caregiver Involvement:

Welcome caregivers to join the yoga practice, fostering a sense of connection between toddlers and their loved ones.

Simple Partner Poses:

Explore simple partner poses where toddlers and caregivers mirror each other's movements. This creates a bonding experience and enhances the sense of security.

8. **Mindful Moments for Toddlers:**

Sensory Exploration:

Incorporate mindful moments through sensory exploration. Introduce textures, scents, or simple tactile activities that engage toddlers' senses during the practice.

Gentle Guided Relaxation:

End the session with a brief guided relaxation, using soft language and soothing imagery to help toddlers wind down.

9. Flexibility and Adaptability:

Embrace Flexibility:

Recognize that toddlers may have varying attention spans and energy levels. Be flexible in adapting the practice based on their cues and interests.

Open Exploration Time:

Allow for open exploration time where toddlers can move freely and express themselves. This unstructured play fosters creativity and a sense of autonomy.

10. Encouraging Expression and Communication:

Creative Expression:

Facilitate creative expression through movement. Encourage toddlers to use their bodies to express emotions or imitate animals, fostering a sense of self-discovery.

Interactive Communication:

Use simple language and interactive communication to guide the practice. Encourage toddlers to share their experiences and observations during and after the session.

11. Community and Social Interaction:

Group Activities:

Organize group activities that promote social interaction. Circle time, where toddlers share a movement or pose with others, fosters a sense of community.

Sharing and Cooperation:

Introduce activities that involve sharing and cooperation, emphasizing the joy of working together. This supports the development of social skills and a positive group dynamic.

12. Safety and Well-being:

Supervision and Support:

Prioritize safety by ensuring adequate supervision during the toddler yoga session. Encourage caregivers to actively participate and provide support as needed.

Adapting for Individual Needs:

Recognize and adapt the practice for individual needs, considering factors like developmental stages, physical abilities, and any specific considerations or sensitivities.

Celebrating Playful Exploration:

Conclude the session by celebrating the toddlers' playful exploration and participation. Emphasize the joy and positive experiences created through the practice.

Invitation for Continued Exploration:

Encourage caregivers to continue exploring yoga with toddlers at home, incorporating elements of play, movement, and connection into their daily routines.

Tailoring yoga practices for toddlers is a delightful adventure that blends movement, imagination, and the inherent joy of discovery. By embracing the unique qualities of this age group and fostering an environment of playfulness, caregivers and yoga instructors create a foundation for positive experiences that support toddlers' physical and emotional development.

6.2 Engaging Yoga for School-age Children

The school-age years mark a period of boundless energy, curiosity, and rapid development. Introducing yoga to school-age children is an opportunity to foster physical well-being, enhance focus, and provide tools for stress management. This section explores strategies and practices to create engaging and age-appropriate yoga experiences for school-age children, transforming the mat into a space of exploration and self-discovery.

1. **Understanding School-Age Development:**

Physical and Cognitive Milestones:

Recognize the physical and cognitive milestones typical of school-age children. Tailor yoga practices to support their evolving abilities and interests.

Social and Emotional Growth:

Acknowledge the importance of social and emotional growth during this stage, integrating practices that promote self-awareness, empathy, and positive communication.

2. **Creating a Positive Yoga Environment:**

Welcoming and Inclusive Space:

Establish a welcoming and inclusive environment that encourages children to express themselves freely. Use colorful mats, props, and age-appropriate decor to make the space inviting.

Celebrating Individuality:

Celebrate the individuality of each child, fostering a sense of acceptance and positive self-image within the yoga community.

3. **Dynamic Warm-Up and Energizers:**

Interactive Warm-Up Activities:

Begin sessions with dynamic warm-up activities that involve playful movements. Incorporate games like "Yoga Simon Says" or "Musical Mats" to energize the group.

Energizing Breathing Exercises:

Introduce breathing exercises that invigorate the body and mind. Techniques like "Balloon Breath" or "Dragon Breath" engage children's imagination while promoting focus.

4.   Yoga Poses for School-Age Children:

Themed Pose Exploration:

Explore themed yoga poses that align with children's interests. Incorporate poses inspired by nature, animals, or popular characters to make the practice engaging.

Balance and Coordination Poses:

Introduce balance and coordination poses that challenge and enhance physical skills. Poses like "Tree Pose" or "Warrior III" contribute to strength and body awareness.

5.   Storytelling and Imaginative Journeys:

Narrative Yoga Adventures:

Integrate storytelling into yoga sessions, taking children on imaginative journeys. Create narratives where poses become part of exciting adventures, fostering creativity and enthusiasm.

Interactive Story Participation:

Encourage children to actively participate in the story by embodying characters through yoga poses. This interactive approach enhances engagement and connection.

6. **Music and Movement Integration:**

Upbeat and Fun Music:

Incorporate upbeat and age-appropriate music into the yoga practice. Use music to signal transitions between poses or create a lively atmosphere during dynamic movements.

Dance-Inspired Yoga Sequences:

Infuse dance-inspired sequences into yoga practices. Combine yoga poses with rhythmic movements, allowing children to express themselves through a fusion of yoga and dance.

7. **Mindfulness and Relaxation Techniques:**

Guided Imagery for Relaxation:

Introduce guided imagery to promote relaxation. Use calming scenarios, such as imagining floating on a cloud or resting in a peaceful meadow, to guide children into a state of mindfulness.

Breath Awareness for Focus:

Incorporate breath awareness exercises to enhance focus and concentration. Techniques like "Star Breath" or "Square Breathing" provide tools for self-regulation.

8. Yoga Games and Challenges:

Team-building Yoga Games:

Introduce team-building yoga games that foster cooperation and communication. Games like "Yoga Charades" or "Partner Poses Challenge" encourage teamwork and social interaction.

Yoga Challenges for Fun:

Create playful yoga challenges that allow children to explore their capabilities. Challenges can include holding poses for a certain duration or completing a sequence in creative ways.

9. **Partner and Group Poses:**

Interactive Partner Poses:

Explore interactive partner poses that require cooperation and communication. Partner poses like "Mirror Pose" or "Partner Boat Pose" enhance social connections and trust.

Group Poses for Unity:

Introduce group poses that promote a sense of unity. Encourage children to collaborate in forming shapes or patterns with their bodies, fostering a shared sense of accomplishment.

10. **Creative Expression and Art Integration:**

Art-Inspired Yoga:

Integrate creative expression by combining art and yoga. Allow children to create artwork inspired by their yoga experiences, fostering a connection between movement and self-expression.

Yoga Doodle Sessions:

Incorporate "yoga doodle" sessions where children use markers or crayons to express their feelings and experiences after a yoga practice.

11. Mindful Reflection and Sharing:

Circle Time Reflection:

Conclude sessions with a circle time for mindful reflection. Encourage children to share their experiences, express gratitude, or discuss how certain poses made them feel.

Empathy-Building Discussions:

Facilitate discussions on empathy and kindness, connecting yoga principles to everyday life. Discuss how mindfulness and compassion can positively impact relationships with peers.

12. Yoga Events and Celebrations:

Yoga Days or Festivals:

Organize special yoga events or celebrations within the school community. This can include yoga days, themed yoga festivals, or performances that showcase the children's yoga journey.

Family Yoga Sessions:

Extend the yoga community by inviting families to participate in special sessions. Family yoga fosters connection and provides an opportunity for shared experiences.

13. Integrating Yoga into Academic Learning:

Yoga for Mind-Body Connection:

Advocate for the integration of yoga into academic settings to support the mind-body connection. Highlight the benefits of brief yoga breaks during the school day to enhance focus and concentration.

Yoga for Stress Reduction:

Emphasize the role of yoga in stress reduction for school-age children. Provide resources for teachers to incorporate simple yoga techniques in the classroom as a means of promoting emotional well-being.

14. Building a Yoga Community:

Yoga Clubs or Groups:

Establish yoga clubs or groups within the school community. These clubs can provide a space for children to continue their yoga journey, share experiences, and build lasting connections.

Yoga Ambassadors:

Empower enthusiastic students to become yoga ambassadors, promoting the benefits of yoga within the school. Encourage them to organize events, share their experiences, and inspire others to join the yoga community.

15. Professional Development for Educators:

Yoga Training for Educators:

Offer professional development opportunities for educators to receive basic yoga training. This equips teachers with the knowledge and tools to incorporate yoga into their classrooms.

Creating Yoga-Informed Spaces:

Encourage educators to create yoga-informed spaces within classrooms. Provide resources and guidance on how to integrate mindful practices, breathing exercises, or short movement breaks into daily routines.

Celebrating Growth and Exploration:

Conclude each session by celebrating the growth, exploration, and positive experiences of the school-age children in their yoga journey.

Invitation to Continued Exploration:

Encourage ongoing exploration of yoga, both within and beyond the school setting. Emphasize the lifelong benefits of mindfulness, movement, and self-discovery.

Engaging yoga for school-age children is a dynamic exploration of movement, mindfulness, and self-expression. By tailoring practices to the developmental stage and interests of these young learners, educators and yoga instructors create an environment that nurtures both physical well-being and a lifelong appreciation for the transformative power of yoga.

6.3 Teen Yoga: Navigating Challenges with Mindfulness

The teenage years are a time of dynamic change, self-discovery, and navigating the complexities of adolescence. Teen yoga emerges as a valuable tool to support physical health, emotional well-being, and the development of mindfulness skills. In this section, we delve into the unique considerations of teaching yoga to teenagers, addressing challenges specific to this age group, and fostering a mindful approach that empowers teens on their journey to self-awareness and resilience.

1. **Understanding the Teenage Experience:**

Physical Changes:

Highlight the role of mindful communication in building healthy relationships. Discuss active listening, empathy, and effective expression as tools for positive interaction.

12. Mindful Movement Beyond the Mat:

Mindful Physical Activities:

Encourage teens to extend mindful movement beyond the yoga mat. Explore other physical activities such as hiking, dancing, or team sports as opportunities for mindful engagement.

Mindful Lifestyle Choices:

Discuss the impact of mindful lifestyle choices on overall well-being. Explore topics such as nutrition, sleep, and screen time, emphasizing the connection between lifestyle and mental health.

13. Mindfulness for Academic Success:

Concentration and Focus Practices:

Introduce mindfulness practices that enhance concentration and focus. Techniques like focused breath awareness or mindful study breaks support academic success.

Acknowledge the physical changes that accompany adolescence, recognizing the impact on body image, self-esteem, and overall well-being.

Emotional Rollercoaster:

Understand the emotional rollercoaster of adolescence, where teens navigate identity formation, peer relationships, and increasing independence.

2. Creating a Teen-Friendly Yoga Environment:

Youthful and Inclusive Space:

Establish a space that feels youthful and inclusive, incorporating vibrant colors, comfortable seating, and opportunities for self-expression.

Encouraging Peer Connection:

Foster a sense of community by encouraging peer connections. Group activities and partner poses create a supportive environment where teens can share their yoga journey.

3. **Mindfulness for Stress Management:**

Mindful Awareness Practices:

Introduce mindfulness practices as tools for stress management. Techniques such as mindful breathing, body scans, and guided meditations provide teens with strategies to navigate stressors.

Mindful Movement:

Emphasize mindful movement within yoga poses, encouraging teens to cultivate awareness of their breath, sensations, and emotions during the practice.

4. **Addressing Body Image and Self-Esteem:**

Positive Body Affirmations:

Incorporate positive body affirmations into the yoga practice. Guide teens to appreciate and respect their bodies, fostering a positive relationship with self-image.

Celebrating Strength and Capability:

Focus on poses that celebrate strength and capability rather than appearance. Empower teens to appreciate the functionality of their bodies and the progress they make in their practice.

5. Yoga for Emotional Regulation:

Emotionally Expressive Poses:

Explore emotionally expressive poses that allow teens to release tension and express emotions. Poses like "Child's Pose" or "Twisting Poses" offer a space for emotional release.

Breath-Centered Emotional Regulation:

Teach breath-centered techniques to regulate emotions. Encourage teens to use breath awareness to navigate challenging situations both on and off the mat.

6. Adapting Yoga Philosophy for Teens:

Relevance of Yoga Philosophy:

Discuss the relevance of yoga philosophy in the context of teens' lives. Explore concepts such as mindfulness, non-judgment, and self-compassion, connecting these principles to everyday experiences.

Values and Ethical Guidelines:

Introduce ethical guidelines from yoga philosophy, emphasizing values like kindness, honesty, and respect. Connect these principles to building positive relationships and navigating ethical challenges.

7.   Mindful Movement Sequences:

Sequences for Emotional Release:

Design sequences that facilitate emotional release through mindful movement. Incorporate flowing sequences, dynamic poses, and transitions that encourage a sense of fluidity and release.

Focus on Mind-Body Connection:

Guide teens in maintaining a strong mind-body connection throughout the practice. Use cues that emphasize sensations, breath, and the integration of movement with awareness.

8.   Empowering Teens through Choice:

Pose Variations and Options:

Provide teens with pose variations and options. Empower them to make choices based on their comfort level and individual preferences, fostering a sense of autonomy.

Theme-Based Classes:

Design theme-based classes that align with the interests and concerns of teens. Themes can range from self-empowerment and resilience to managing stress and building positive relationships.

9.   Peer-Supported Yoga Activities:

Group Poses and Challenges:

Introduce group poses and challenges that encourage collaboration and peer support. Activities like partner yoga, group balances, or synchronized movements foster a sense of unity.

Shared Mindfulness Practices:

Facilitate shared mindfulness practices within the group. Group meditation, mindful discussions, or reflective journaling sessions provide opportunities for teens to connect and support each other.

10. Yoga for Building Resilience:

Resilience-Building Poses:

Explore poses that build physical and emotional resilience. Poses such as "Warrior Poses" and inversions symbolize strength and overcoming challenges.

Mindful Coping Strategies:

Teach mindful coping strategies for dealing with setbacks and stress. Discuss the concept of resilience as an adaptive response to adversity, emphasizing the importance of self-care and seeking support.

11. Real-World Application of Mindfulness:

Mindfulness in Daily Life:

Discuss the real-world application of mindfulness in teens' daily lives. Explore how mindfulness can be integrated into school, relationships, and decision-making processes.

Mindful Communication:

Stress Reduction Techniques:

Teach stress reduction techniques that can be applied during exams or challenging academic periods. Mindful breathing, short movement breaks, or visualization exercises offer tools for managing stress.

14. Community-Building Yoga Events:

Teen Yoga Workshops:

Organize teen-specific yoga workshops or events. These gatherings provide a platform for teens to connect, share experiences, and explore yoga in a supportive community.

Teen Yoga Retreats:

Consider organizing teen yoga retreats that offer immersive experiences, fostering deeper connections and providing a space for introspection and growth.

15. Parent and Caregiver Involvement:

Family Yoga Sessions:

Introduce family yoga sessions to involve parents and caregivers. This provides an opportunity for shared experiences and reinforces mindfulness practices within the family unit.

Communication and Support:

Foster open communication with parents and caregivers, providing resources and information on the benefits of teen yoga. Encourage a supportive home environment that reinforces mindfulness principles.

Celebrating Teen Empowerment:

Conclude each session by celebrating the empowerment and self-discovery of teens through yoga. Acknowledge their resilience and commitment to personal growth.

Invitation to Ongoing Mindful Exploration:

Extend an invitation for teens to continue their mindful exploration, both on and off the mat. Emphasize that yoga serves as a lifelong tool for well-being and self-discovery.

Teen yoga becomes a transformative journey that navigates the challenges of adolescence with mindfulness and empowerment. By addressing the unique needs of this age group, yoga instructors create an environment that supports teens in building resilience, cultivating positive relationships, and embracing the transformative power of mindfulness on their path to self-discovery.

Chapter 7: Overcoming Challenges

In the journey of integrating yoga into various aspects of life, challenges inevitably arise. This chapter serves as a guide to navigate and overcome these challenges, offering insights and practical strategies for individuals, instructors, and communities committed to the transformative power of yoga.

1. **Resisting Resistance:**

Understanding Resistance:

Explore the concept of resistance that individuals may face when introduced to yoga. Understand the factors contributing to resistance, such as misconceptions, cultural biases, or unfamiliarity.

Cultivating Openness:

Discuss strategies to cultivate openness and curiosity, emphasizing the diverse benefits of yoga for physical health, mental well-being, and personal growth.

Adapting Approaches:

Provide adaptable approaches for instructors to tailor their teaching methods based on the unique needs and concerns of individuals resistant to yoga.

2. Inclusivity and Accessibility:

Cultural Sensitivity:

Address the importance of cultural sensitivity in yoga practices, acknowledging diverse backgrounds, beliefs, and traditions.

Adapting for Special Populations:

Discuss strategies for adapting yoga practices to make them accessible and inclusive for special populations, including individuals with disabilities, chronic illnesses, or specific health conditions.

Creating Inclusive Spaces:

Advocate for the creation of inclusive yoga spaces that welcome practitioners of all abilities and backgrounds, fostering a sense of belonging.

3. **Time Constraints and Busy Lifestyles:**

Short Yoga Practices:

Introduce the concept of short and effective yoga practices for individuals with busy schedules. Highlight the benefits of incorporating brief sessions into daily routines for physical and mental well-being.

Creating Consistent Habits:

Provide tips for creating consistent yoga habits, emphasizing the integration of yoga into daily life as a manageable and sustainable practice.

Online Resources for Flexibility:

Explore the flexibility offered by online resources, enabling individuals to access yoga classes and guided practices at their convenience.

4. **Financial Barriers:**

Affordable Alternatives:

Address financial barriers to yoga participation by highlighting affordable alternatives. Discuss community classes, online platforms with free content, and low-cost resources to make yoga accessible to a wider audience.

Community Support Programs:

Advocate for community support programs that offer subsidized or free yoga classes, promoting inclusivity and ensuring that financial constraints do not hinder access to the benefits of yoga.

DIY Home Practices:

Encourage individuals to explore do-it-yourself (DIY) home practices, using minimal equipment and resources. Provide guidance on creating a supportive home environment for yoga.

5. Maintaining Motivation:

Setting Realistic Goals:

Discuss the importance of setting realistic and achievable goals in maintaining motivation for a consistent yoga practice. Emphasize the gradual progression and the celebration of small milestones.

Variety in Practices:

Introduce variety in yoga practices to keep individuals engaged. Explore different styles, themes, and approaches to cater to diverse interests and preferences.

Mindful Reflection:

Guide individuals in practicing mindful reflection, encouraging them to recognize and appreciate the positive changes and benefits that arise from their yoga journey.

6. **Injury Prevention and Recovery:**

Understanding Physical Limits:

Emphasize the significance of understanding and respecting physical limits to prevent injuries. Provide guidance on proper alignment, modification of poses, and the importance of listening to the body.

Yoga as a Healing Tool:

Highlight the therapeutic aspects of yoga for injury recovery. Discuss gentle and restorative practices that support healing and rehabilitation while maintaining a connection to the practice.

Consulting Healthcare Professionals:

Encourage individuals to consult healthcare professionals, particularly when dealing with pre-existing conditions or injuries. Stress the importance of seeking guidance for a safe and personalized yoga practice.

7.   Online Yoga Etiquette:

Respecting Virtual Spaces:

Discuss the etiquette of participating in online yoga classes, emphasizing the importance of creating a respectful and focused virtual environment.

Engaging Responsibly:

Guide individuals in engaging responsibly during online classes, including muting microphones when necessary, using appropriate video settings, and respecting the privacy of others.

Effective Communication:

Explore effective communication in virtual yoga spaces, fostering a sense of community despite physical distance. Discuss ways to ask questions, provide feedback, and connect with instructors and fellow practitioners.

8. **Social Stigma and Misconceptions:**

Addressing Misconceptions:

Address common misconceptions and social stigmas associated with yoga. Provide accurate information about the diverse nature of yoga, dispelling myths that may discourage individuals from engaging in the practice.

Community Awareness Campaigns:

Advocate for community awareness campaigns to promote a broader understanding of yoga and its inclusive nature. Emphasize the diverse benefits beyond the physical aspects, including mental health and well-being.

Personal Testimonials:

Share personal testimonials from individuals who have experienced positive transformations through yoga. Highlight diverse stories to showcase the inclusivity and adaptability of yoga for various lifestyles and backgrounds.

9.   **Lack of Supportive Communities:**

Building Supportive Networks:

Guide individuals in building supportive yoga communities, both online and offline. Discuss the benefits of connecting with like-minded individuals, sharing experiences, and fostering a sense of belonging.

Community-led Initiatives:

Encourage community-led initiatives to create supportive spaces for yoga practitioners. Discuss the potential of grassroots efforts, local events, or online forums that facilitate connections and mutual support.

Promoting Inclusivity:

Stress the importance of promoting inclusivity within yoga communities. Advocate for welcoming environments that embrace diversity, celebrate individual journeys, and encourage collaboration.

10.   **Maintaining a Lifelong Practice:**

Adapting to Life Changes:

Discuss strategies for adapting yoga practices to accommodate life changes, such as parenthood, career shifts, or aging. Emphasize the flexibility of yoga as a lifelong companion that evolves with individuals.

Integrating Yoga into Daily Rituals:

Explore the integration of yoga into daily rituals, emphasizing its role as a grounding and centering practice amidst life's fluctuations.

Continued Learning and Exploration:

Encourage a mindset of continued learning and exploration. Discuss the richness of the yoga journey and the potential for deepening the practice through ongoing education, workshops, and exposure to diverse styles.

Empowering Through Challenges:

Conclude the chapter by emphasizing the empowerment that arises from navigating and overcoming challenges in the yoga journey.

Invitation to Resilience:

Extend an invitation for individuals, instructors, and communities to approach challenges with resilience, adaptability, and a commitment to the transformative power of yoga.

Overcoming challenges in the realm of yoga becomes an integral part of the transformative journey. By addressing resistance, fostering inclusivity, and providing practical strategies, individuals can navigate hurdles, ensuring that yoga remains a source of empowerment and well-being for everyone.

7.1 Addressing Common Concerns in Kids' Yoga

Embarking on the journey of teaching yoga to children is a rewarding endeavor, but it comes with its own set of common concerns. This section aims to address these concerns and provide insights for parents, caregivers, and instructors to create a positive and enriching kids' yoga experience.

1. **Safety First:**

Instructor Qualifications:

Address concerns about the qualifications of yoga instructors working with children. Emphasize the importance of certified instructors with specialized training in kids' yoga, including child development and safety protocols.

Supervision and Class Ratios:

Highlight the significance of adequate supervision and appropriate class ratios. Ensuring that there is a proper balance between instructors to children promotes a safe and supportive environment.

2. Physical Development and Capabilities:

Age-Appropriate Practices:

Alleviate concerns regarding age-appropriate practices. Emphasize that kids' yoga is designed to accommodate varying physical abilities and developmental stages, providing modifications for different age groups.

Encouraging Individual Progress:

Communicate the focus on individual progress rather than comparison. Kids' yoga celebrates each child's unique development and encourages self-expression in a non-competitive setting.

3. Mindfulness and Attention Span:

Introduction to Mindfulness:

Address concerns about introducing mindfulness practices to children. Explain that kids' yoga incorporates playful and engaging mindfulness activities designed to align with their natural curiosity and shorter attention spans.

Interactive and Dynamic Sessions:

Emphasize the use of interactive and dynamic sessions to maintain children's interest. Incorporate games, storytelling, and thematic elements that capture their imagination and foster mindfulness in a fun way.

4.   Ensuring Engagement:

Varied and Interactive Content:

Acknowledge concerns about keeping children engaged. Highlight the importance of varied and interactive content, including age-appropriate yoga poses, creative movement, and games that make the experience enjoyable.

Incorporating Playfulness:

Emphasize the playfulness inherent in kids' yoga. Encourage instructors to infuse humor, storytelling, and imaginative elements into the sessions to create an engaging and enjoyable atmosphere.

5.   Communication with Parents:

Transparent Communication:

Address concerns related to communication with parents. Advocate for transparent communication between instructors and parents, sharing insights into class activities, learning objectives, and any notable observations about the child's participation.

Open Channels for Feedback:

Establish open channels for feedback from parents. Encourage parents to share their concerns, preferences, and insights to create a collaborative and supportive environment.

6. Integration into School Curriculum:

Educational Benefits:

Address concerns about the integration of kids' yoga into the school curriculum. Highlight the educational benefits, including improved focus, stress reduction, and enhanced physical coordination, which contribute to overall well-being.

Collaboration with Educators:

Advocate for collaboration between yoga instructors and educators. Emphasize the potential for kids' yoga to complement academic learning and contribute to a positive school environment.

7. Cultural Sensitivity:

Respecting Diverse Backgrounds:

Address concerns related to cultural sensitivity in kids' yoga. Emphasize the importance of respecting diverse backgrounds and beliefs, while ensuring that yoga practices are presented in an inclusive and culturally sensitive manner.

Choosing Inclusive Themes:

Encourage instructors to choose inclusive themes that resonate with a broad range of cultural experiences. This approach fosters a sense of unity and belonging among children from various backgrounds.

8. Creating a Positive Environment:

Nurturing Inclusivity:

Address concerns about creating a positive and inclusive environment. Emphasize the importance of nurturing inclusivity, where all children feel welcome, valued, and encouraged to express themselves freely.

Anti-Bullying Policies:

Advocate for the implementation of anti-bullying policies within kids' yoga programs. Emphasize the role of instructors and caregivers in fostering a supportive and respectful atmosphere.

9. Incorporating Technology:

Balancing Screen Time:

Address concerns related to incorporating technology into kids' yoga. Emphasize the need for a balanced approach, using technology as a supplementary tool for virtual classes or resources while prioritizing in-person interaction and movement.

Parental Consent and Privacy:

Highlight the importance of obtaining parental consent for any use of technology in kids' yoga programs. Emphasize the protection of children's privacy and adherence to online safety guidelines.

10. Managing Diverse Abilities:

Adapting Practices:

Acknowledge concerns about managing diverse abilities among children. Emphasize the adaptability of kids' yoga practices, providing modifications and variations to accommodate individual needs.

Encouraging Inclusivity:

Foster a culture of inclusivity where children of all abilities feel comfortable participating. Encourage instructors to be mindful of diverse needs and create an environment that promotes collaboration and support.

Collaborative Approach:

Conclude this section by emphasizing a collaborative approach among parents, caregivers, and instructors to address concerns and create a positive and enriching kids' yoga experience.

Continuous Communication:

Encourage continuous communication to ensure that any concerns are promptly addressed, and that the kids' yoga journey remains a joyful and beneficial experience for all involved.

Navigating concerns in kids' yoga involves a collaborative effort to prioritize safety, inclusivity, and engaging practices. By addressing these common concerns, parents, caregivers, and instructors contribute to creating a positive and enriching environment where children can thrive on their yoga journey.

7.2 Adapting Yoga for Children with Special Needs

Teaching yoga to children with special needs requires a thoughtful and inclusive approach that recognizes and honors each child's unique abilities. This section provides insights and practical guidance for yoga instructors, parents, and caregivers, emphasizing the adaptability of yoga to create a supportive and enriching experience for children with diverse needs.

1.   **Understanding Individual Needs:**

Holistic Assessment:

Emphasize the importance of a holistic assessment to understand each child's unique abilities, challenges, and preferences. Consider physical, sensory, cognitive, and emotional factors when tailoring yoga practices.

Communication with Caregivers:

Advocate for open communication with caregivers to gather valuable insights into a child's medical history, sensory sensitivities, and any specific instructions or modifications needed.

2.   **Creating an Inclusive Environment:**

Welcoming and Supportive Atmosphere:

Establish a welcoming and supportive atmosphere in the yoga space. Ensure that the environment is sensory-friendly, free from excessive stimuli, and equipped with necessary accommodations for children with diverse needs.

Inclusive Language and Instructions:

Use inclusive language and instructions that resonate with all children. Provide clear, simple, and visual cues to enhance understanding, and be mindful of each child's communication style and preferences.

3. **Tailoring Asanas and Sequences:**

Modified Poses for Comfort:

Modify yoga poses to accommodate individual comfort levels and physical abilities. Focus on poses that enhance flexibility, strength, and body awareness while respecting each child's range of motion.

Sequencing for Flow and Stability:

Create sequences that promote flow and stability. Emphasize smooth transitions between poses, allowing children with special needs to engage in movements that enhance both physical and emotional well-being.

4.   **Sensory Integration Techniques:**

Mindful Sensory Exploration:

Incorporate sensory integration techniques into yoga practices. Engage children in mindful sensory exploration, such as feeling different textures, using sensory-friendly props, or incorporating calming scents to enhance the overall experience.

Breath Awareness for Self-Regulation:

Introduce breath awareness exercises as tools for self-regulation. Teach children how mindful breathing can help manage sensory overload, anxiety, or stress, fostering a sense of control.

5.   **Adapting Mindfulness Practices:**

Gentle Mindfulness Techniques:

Adapt mindfulness practices to suit each child's needs. Introduce gentle mindfulness techniques, such as guided imagery, soft music, or mindful coloring, to create a calming and centered experience.

Encouraging Mindful Expression:

Encourage mindful expression through movement, allowing children to explore their emotions through yoga. Provide opportunities for creative expression, such as dance-inspired movements or simple, expressive yoga sequences.

6. Incorporating Therapeutic Tools:

Yoga Props for Support:

Utilize therapeutic tools and props to provide additional support. Bolsters, blankets, and straps can enhance comfort and stability, especially during seated or reclined poses.

Visual Aids and Storytelling:

Integrate visual aids and storytelling to enhance engagement. Use visuals, social stories, or picture schedules to help children understand and navigate the structure of the yoga session.

7. Building Trust and Connection:

Establishing a Personal Connection:

Prioritize building a personal connection with each child. Establish trust through positive reinforcement, encouragement, and adapting teaching approaches to align with the child's comfort level.

Consistency in Practices:

Maintain consistency in yoga practices to create a sense of predictability and security. Consistent routines and familiar activities contribute to a more comfortable and enjoyable experience for children with special needs.

8.   Collaboration with Caregivers:

Involvement in Yoga Practices:

Encourage caregivers to participate in yoga practices when appropriate. Their involvement not only provides additional support but also allows them to learn and practice adapted techniques that can be beneficial outside of the yoga sessions.

Open Communication Channels:

Establish open communication channels with caregivers to share progress, challenges, and modifications. Collaborate on strategies that can be implemented both in the yoga setting and at home.

9.   Promoting Social Interaction:

Group Activities with Sensitivity:

Include group activities with sensitivity to social dynamics. Foster a supportive atmosphere that encourages social interaction, understanding, and acceptance among children with and without special needs.

Buddy Systems and Peer Support:

Implement buddy systems or peer support structures, where children can pair up to provide assistance and companionship. This approach promotes inclusivity and a sense of community within the yoga class.

10. Professional Development for Instructors:

Specialized Training Opportunities:

Advocate for specialized training opportunities for yoga instructors working with children with special needs. These training programs should cover inclusive teaching methods, adaptive practices, and strategies for creating an accessible and supportive yoga environment.

Continual Learning and Collaboration:

Promote continual learning and collaboration among yoga instructors, therapists, and educators. Encourage the sharing of insights, resources, and best practices to enhance the collective knowledge in adapting yoga for children with diverse needs.

11. Celebrating Achievements:

Acknowledging Individual Progress:

Acknowledge and celebrate each child's individual progress and achievements. Emphasize the importance of recognizing milestones, no matter how small, as they contribute to the child's overall well-being and sense of accomplishment.

Inclusive Recognition Practices:

Implement inclusive recognition practices within the class. This may include certificates, positive affirmations, or collaborative activities that highlight the unique strengths and contributions of each child.

12. Advocating for Inclusivity:

Raising Awareness in the Community:

Advocate for inclusivity and raise awareness in the broader community. Promote understanding and acceptance of diverse abilities, emphasizing the transformative benefits of adapted yoga practices for children with special needs.

Community Events and Workshops:

Organize community events or workshops that showcase inclusive yoga practices. Provide opportunities for families, caregivers, and community members to participate and learn about the positive impact of adapted yoga for children with diverse needs.

Empowering Through Adaptation:

Conclude this section by highlighting the empowerment that comes through the adaptation of yoga for children with special needs. By embracing inclusivity, understanding individual needs, and fostering a supportive environment, yoga becomes a transformative and enriching experience for every child.

Adapting yoga for children with special needs is a journey of compassion, creativity, and inclusion. Through thoughtful modifications and a commitment to individualized support, yoga becomes a powerful tool for promoting physical, emotional, and social well-being in every child, regardless of their unique abilities.

7.3 Building a Supportive Community for Kids' Yoga

Creating a supportive community for kids' yoga goes beyond the confines of the yoga mat. It involves fostering connections among parents, caregivers, instructors, and the broader community to create an environment where children can thrive physically, mentally, and emotionally. In this section, we explore key strategies and initiatives to build a strong and inclusive community around kids' yoga.

1. **Parent and Caregiver Involvement:**

Family Yoga Sessions:

Introduce family yoga sessions to involve parents and caregivers. These sessions provide an opportunity for shared experiences and reinforce mindfulness practices within the family unit.

Communication Channels:

Establish clear communication channels with parents and caregivers. Regular updates, newsletters, and information sharing create a sense of transparency and keep families informed about the benefits and activities of kids' yoga.

2. **Community Workshops and Events:**

Educational Workshops:

Organize educational workshops on the benefits of kids' yoga. Address common questions, share insights into the positive impact on child development, and provide practical tips for incorporating yoga into daily routines.

Community Events:

Host community events that celebrate the joy of kids' yoga. Fun gatherings, themed events, or outdoor yoga picnics create opportunities for families to connect and form lasting bonds.

3. Online Platforms for Connection:

Virtual Community Spaces:

Establish virtual community spaces for parents, caregivers, and instructors. Online forums, social media groups, or dedicated platforms facilitate communication, resource sharing, and the exchange of ideas.

Webinars and Q&A Sessions:

Conduct webinars and Q&A sessions to provide valuable information and address concerns. This interactive approach fosters a sense of community engagement and allows participants to connect with experts and fellow community members.

4. Community Outreach Programs:

School and Community Partnerships:

Forge partnerships with schools and community organizations to integrate kids' yoga into broader educational initiatives. Collaborate on wellness programs, after-school activities, or community outreach events to expand the reach of yoga practices.

Volunteer Opportunities:

Offer volunteer opportunities for community members to get involved. This could include assisting in classes, organizing events, or contributing to outreach programs that make kids' yoga accessible to a wider audience.

5. **Supportive Networks for Instructors:**

Professional Development Workshops:

Host professional development workshops for kids' yoga instructors. These workshops can focus on inclusive teaching methods, adapting practices for diverse needs, and creating a supportive and positive class environment.

Peer Support Groups:

Establish peer support groups for instructors to connect, share experiences, and exchange ideas. These groups provide a platform for collaboration, mentorship, and continual learning within the community.

6. Cultivating a Positive Atmosphere:

Positive Communication Practices:

Foster positive communication practices within the community. Encourage the use of affirming language, constructive feedback, and expressions of gratitude to create a supportive and uplifting atmosphere.

Celebrating Achievements:

Celebrate the achievements of children, parents, and instructors within the community. Recognition ceremonies, achievement boards, or simple acknowledgments contribute to a culture of positivity and encouragement.

7. Community-Based Challenges and Initiatives:

Yoga Challenges for Families:

Launch community-based yoga challenges for families. These challenges, whether in person or online, encourage participation, create a sense of camaraderie, and showcase the diverse ways families incorporate yoga into their lives.

Charity and Outreach Initiatives:

Organize charity and outreach initiatives that connect kids' yoga with community service. Events such as charity yoga classes or partnerships with local organizations emphasize the broader impact of yoga beyond individual well-being.

8. **Inclusive Language and Representation:**

The language that Fosters Inclusivity:

Use language that fosters inclusivity in all communications. Ensure that promotional materials, class instructions, and community messages are reflective of diverse backgrounds, abilities, and family structures.

Representation in Visuals:

Include diverse representations in visual materials. This extends to images, posters, and online content, reinforcing a sense of belonging for all families and children in the community.

9. **Feedback and Continuous Improvement:**

Feedback Mechanisms:

Establish feedback mechanisms to gather insights from the community. Surveys, suggestion boxes, or regular feedback sessions provide valuable information for continuous improvement and tailoring kids' yoga programs to community needs.

Adapting Programs Based on Feedback:

Actively adapt kids' yoga programs based on community feedback. This responsiveness demonstrates a commitment to meeting the evolving needs of families and ensures that the community remains an integral part of the decision-making process.

10. Collaborative Events with Local Businesses:

Partnerships with Local Businesses:

Collaborate with local businesses to host collaborative events. Partnering with wellness-oriented businesses, bookstores, or recreational venues can create a network of support for kids' yoga and introduce families to a range of well-being resources.

Discounts and Promotions:

Negotiate discounts or promotions with local businesses for community members. This could include discounts on yoga props, wellness services, or family-friendly activities, enhancing the value of being part of the kids' yoga community.

11. Embracing Diversity and Inclusion:

Diverse Programming and Themes:

Embrace diversity in programming and themes. Ensure that kids' yoga classes incorporate diverse cultural elements, celebrations, and traditions, fostering an inclusive environment that respects and appreciates differences.

Celebrating Cultural Awareness:

Celebrate cultural awareness within the community. Organize events or workshops that promote understanding, educate about different cultures, and celebrate the rich tapestry of diversity within the kids' yoga community.

12. Inclusive Policies and Accessibility:

Accessible Class Options:

Offer accessible class options to accommodate various schedules and needs. This may include a mix of in-person, virtual, or recorded classes to ensure flexibility and inclusivity for all community members.

Financial Accessibility:

Implement financial accessibility policies. Consider sliding scale fees, scholarships, or community-funded programs to ensure that financial constraints do not hinder access to kids' yoga for families in need.

Nurturing a Flourishing Community:

Conclude this section by highlighting the collective effort in nurturing a flourishing community for kids' yoga. By fostering connections, embracing diversity, and prioritizing inclusivity, the community becomes a supportive and enriching space for the growth and well-being of every child.

Building a supportive community for kids' yoga is a collaborative journey that involves the active participation of parents, caregivers, instructors, and the broader community. Through intentional efforts to connect, communicate, and celebrate together, this community becomes a vibrant source of support, encouragement, and joy for children and their families on their yoga journey.

Chapter 8: The Journey Continues

As we embark on the concluding chapter of "Yoga for Kids: The Ultimate Guide to Yoga for Bend, Breathe, and Grow with Empowering Children through Mindfulness, Flexibility, and Fun with Yoga," we find ourselves at a juncture where the journey of discovery, growth, and well-being continues. This chapter serves as a reflection on the transformative power of yoga for children and an invitation for the journey to extend beyond the pages of this guide.

1. Reflections on Growth:

Celebrating Progress:

Take a moment to celebrate the progress made on the yoga journey. Reflect on the physical, mental, and emotional growth that children have experienced through the empowering practices of yoga.

Notable Achievements:

Highlight notable achievements, whether they be mastering a challenging pose, cultivating mindfulness, or expressing creativity through movement. Recognize the resilience and dedication that children have demonstrated along the way.

2. Empowering Through Mindfulness:

Mindfulness as a Lifelong Skill:

Emphasize the enduring nature of mindfulness as a lifelong skill. Discuss how the mindfulness techniques learned in kids' yoga serve as valuable tools for navigating challenges, fostering resilience, and enhancing overall well-being.

Encouragement for Continued Mindful Practices:

Encourage children, parents, and caregivers to continue integrating mindfulness into daily life. Whether through brief moments of mindful breathing, gratitude practices, or awareness of the present moment, mindfulness becomes a lifelong companion.

3. Building Resilience:

Yoga as a Resilience Builder:

Explore the role of yoga in building resilience. Discuss how the physical and mental aspects of yoga contribute to resilience, teaching children to bounce back from setbacks, adapt to change, and face life's challenges with a sense of inner strength.

Narratives of Resilience:

Share narratives of resilience, drawing inspiration from real-life stories of individuals who have faced adversity and found strength through yoga. These stories serve as beacons of hope and encouragement for the ongoing journey.

4. Cultivating a Lifelong Practice:

Yoga as a Lifelong Companion:

Discuss the idea of yoga as a lifelong companion. Emphasize that the practices learned in childhood evolve and adapt, becoming a source of support, self-discovery, and well-being throughout various stages of life.

Exploration of Advanced Practices:

Invite those who have engaged with kids' yoga to explore advanced practices, styles, or specialized areas of interest within the broader field of yoga. This continued exploration ensures that the journey remains dynamic and enriching.

5. Community and Connection:

Sustaining Community Bonds:

Reflect on the importance of sustaining community bonds formed through kids' yoga. Encourage ongoing participation in community events, workshops, and collaborative initiatives that strengthen the sense of connection and support.

Stories of Community Impact:

Share stories of community impact, highlighting instances where the collective efforts of families, caregivers, and instructors have made a positive difference in the lives of children. These stories inspire a sense of shared purpose and connection.

6. Gratitude for the Journey:

Expressions of Gratitude:

Express gratitude for the journey. Acknowledge the dedication of parents, caregivers, and instructors who have played a pivotal role in fostering a positive and empowering environment for children to thrive.

Children's Expressions of Gratitude:

Showcase expressions of gratitude from children. Whether through artwork, written reflections, or verbal testimonials, children's voices contribute to the tapestry of gratitude woven throughout the kids' yoga community.

7. Looking Ahead:

Anticipation for Future Growth:

Anticipate future growth on the yoga journey. Discuss the exciting possibilities and potential avenues for expansion, innovation, and the continuous evolution of kids' yoga practices.

Incorporating Feedback and Insights:

Encourage the community to share feedback and insights for the future. Emphasize the collaborative nature of the journey, where the collective wisdom and experiences of individuals contribute to the ongoing refinement of kids' yoga programs.

8. Invitation to Share the Journey:

Sharing Personal Stories:

Extend an invitation for individuals to share their personal stories of growth and transformation through kids' yoga. Whether through written testimonials, videos, or creative expressions, these shared narratives become a source of inspiration for others.

#YogaForKidsJourney:

Introduce a social media campaign, such as #YogaForKidsJourney, where individuals can share their kids' yoga experiences, achievements, and moments of joy. This collective sharing creates a digital community that extends the reach and impact of the kids' yoga journey.

A Continual Path of Growth:

Conclude the chapter by emphasizing that the journey of kids' yoga is a continual path of growth, exploration, and empowerment. The practices learned, the connections formed, and the resilience cultivated contribute to a holistic approach to well-being that extends far beyond the mat.

Gratitude for Being Part of the Journey:

Express gratitude for being part of the kids' yoga journey. Whether as a parent, caregiver, instructor, or community member, each individual plays a vital role in shaping an environment where children can bend, breathe, and grow with the transformative power of yoga.

As the journey continues, may the empowering practices of kids' yoga ripple through the lives of children, families, and communities, fostering a culture of well-being, mindfulness, and joy. The concluding chapter invites everyone to embrace the ongoing adventure, celebrating the profound impact of kids' yoga on the lives it touches.

8.1 Lifelong Benefits of Kids' Yoga

The practice of yoga among children extends far beyond the playful movements on a mat; it lays the foundation for a lifetime of holistic well-being. From physical flexibility to emotional resilience, the benefits of kids' yoga are multifaceted, shaping individuals into mindful, adaptable, and balanced adults. This section explores the enduring advantages that children carry with them throughout their lives as a result of engaging in yoga from an early age.

1. **Physical Well-Being:**

Flexibility and Strength:

The flexibility and strength cultivated through kids' yoga endure into adulthood. Limbs that are nimble, joints that move with ease, and a foundation of strength become lifelong assets, promoting overall physical well-being.

Healthy Posture and Alignment:

The focus on proper alignment and posture in kids' yoga contributes to a lifetime of musculoskeletal health. Children who develop awareness of their bodies maintain good posture, reducing the risk of chronic conditions associated with poor alignment.

2. Emotional Resilience:

Stress Management:

Mindfulness practices learned in kids' yoga become tools for stress management in adulthood. The ability to navigate challenges with a calm mind and resilient spirit contributes to emotional well-being throughout life.

Emotional Intelligence:

Kids' yoga fosters emotional intelligence, allowing individuals to recognize, understand, and manage their emotions. This lifelong skill enhances interpersonal relationships, communication, and the ability to navigate complex social dynamics.

3. Mindfulness Practices:

Mindful Living:

The foundation of mindfulness laid in childhood extends into adult life. Individuals who are introduced to mindful breathing, awareness, and presence in kids' yoga carry these practices into their daily lives, promoting a sense of centeredness and mindfulness in various situations.

Stress Reduction:

The mindfulness techniques acquired through kids' yoga serve as effective stress-reduction tools. Adults who continue to incorporate mindfulness into their routines experience reduced stress levels, improved mental clarity, and an enhanced ability to respond to challenges with composure.

4. Healthy Lifestyle Choices:

Inclination towards Physical Activity:

Children who engage in yoga are more likely to maintain an inclination towards physical activity as adults. The positive associations with movement and well-being established in childhood contribute to a lifelong commitment to staying active.

Balanced Nutrition and Self-Care:

The holistic approach of kids' yoga extends beyond physical activity to encompass balanced nutrition and self-care practices. Individuals raised with an awareness of the mind-body connection are more likely to make choices that support their overall well-being.

5.   Cultivation of Creativity:

Innovative Thinking:

The creative and imaginative aspects of kids' yoga lay the groundwork for innovative thinking in adulthood. Individuals who are encouraged to express themselves creatively on the mat often become innovative thinkers, problem solvers, and individuals who approach challenges with a creative mindset.

Artistic Expression:

The connection between movement and artistic expression established in kids' yoga may lead to a lifelong affinity for creative outlets. Adults who explore activities such as dance, art, or writing may find these to be essential tools for self-expression and stress relief.

6.   Social Connection and Empathy:

Positive Relationship Building:

Kids' yoga emphasizes positive social interaction and cooperation. Adults who experienced this emphasis in their formative years tend to excel in building and maintaining positive relationships, contributing to a strong support network throughout life.

Empathy and Compassion:

The focus on empathy and compassion in kids' yoga fosters a lifelong commitment to understanding and supporting others. Individuals who develop these qualities in childhood contribute positively to their communities and create a ripple effect of kindness.

7. Self-Discovery and Confidence:

Authentic Self-Expression:

Kids' yoga encourages authentic self-expression and self-discovery. Adults who were given the space to explore their identities on the mat often carry this sense of authenticity into their adult lives, fostering confidence in expressing their true selves.

Resilient Self-Image:

A positive self-image cultivated through kids' yoga remains a lifelong asset. Individuals who learn to appreciate their bodies, minds, and unique qualities are more likely to navigate life's challenges with resilience and a sense of self-worth.

8. Calm and Focused Mind:

Enhanced Concentration:

The mindfulness practices in kids' yoga contribute to enhanced concentration and focus. Adults who carry this ability into their professional and personal lives find themselves better equipped to tackle tasks, make decisions, and maintain a sense of clarity amidst life's complexities.

Stress Reduction in Adulthood:

The stress-reducing benefits of a calm and focused mind persist into adulthood. Individuals who learn to manage stress through kids' yoga are more likely to apply these skills in the workplace, relationships, and daily challenges.

9.   **Adaptability and Open-Mindedness:**

Resilience to Change:

Kids' yoga teaches adaptability and open-mindedness to new experiences. Adults who internalize these principles are more resilient in the face of change, fostering a positive approach to evolving circumstances and a willingness to embrace new opportunities.

Cultivation of Curiosity:

The cultivation of curiosity in kids' yoga encourages a lifelong desire for learning and exploration. Adults who maintain a curious mindset tend to approach life with enthusiasm, adaptability, and a continuous thirst for knowledge.

10. Contribution to a Balanced Lifestyle:

Holistic Approach to Well-Being:

The holistic approach of kids' yoga sets the stage for a balanced lifestyle. Adults who embrace this philosophy prioritize not only physical fitness but also mental, emotional, and spiritual well-being, leading to a more fulfilled and harmonious life.

Integration into Daily Routines:

The integration of yoga practices into daily routines established in childhood becomes a lifelong commitment. Adults who dedicate time to yoga find that it becomes a cornerstone of their self-care regimen, contributing to overall health and longevity.

A Lifelong Journey of Well-Being:

Conclude this section by emphasizing that the benefits of kids' yoga extend far beyond childhood, shaping individuals into well-rounded, resilient, and mindful adults. The practices learned on the mat become integral components of a lifelong journey toward holistic well-being.

Gratitude for the Gift of Yoga:

Express gratitude for the gift of yoga, recognizing its transformative power in fostering a lifetime of physical, mental, and emotional health. Encourage individuals to carry the lessons learned in kids' yoga as enduring tools for navigating the journey of life.

The lifelong benefits of kids' yoga create a lasting legacy of well-being, resilience, and mindfulness. As children grow into adults, the positive imprint of their early yoga experiences becomes a guiding force, influencing their choices, perspectives, and overall quality of life.

9.2 Encouraging a Continued Yoga Practice

Embarking on a journey of yoga is not just a momentary endeavor; it is a lifelong commitment to well-being, mindfulness, and self-discovery. As individuals transition from childhood through adolescence and into adulthood, the encouragement to sustain a yoga practice remains pivotal. This section offers guidance on fostering a continued and meaningful yoga practice, ensuring that the transformative benefits of yoga endure throughout various stages of life.

Setting Realistic and Sustainable Goals:

1. **Reflecting on Personal Objectives:**

Encourage individuals to reflect on their personal objectives for practicing yoga. Whether it's physical fitness, stress management, or spiritual growth, understanding one's goals sets the foundation for a tailored and sustainable yoga practice.

2.   Setting Realistic Milestones:

Emphasize the importance of setting realistic and achievable milestones. Gradual progress, celebrated through small victories, fosters a sense of accomplishment and motivates individuals to persist in their yoga journey.

Diversifying Yoga Practices:

Exploring Different Yoga Styles:

Advocate for the exploration of various yoga styles. From Hatha and Vinyasa to Yin and Kundalini, diversifying yoga practices introduces novelty, prevents monotony, and allows individuals to discover the styles that resonate most with their preferences and needs.

Incorporating Mindfulness Techniques:

Highlight the integration of mindfulness techniques beyond the physical postures. Incorporating meditation, breathwork, and mindfulness exercises enriches the overall yoga experience, offering a holistic approach that aligns with different stages of life.

3. Adapting to Changing Life Circumstances:

Yoga as a Flexible Companion:

Frame yoga as a flexible companion that adapts to changing life circumstances. Emphasize that yoga can be tailored to suit different schedules, physical conditions, and life transitions, ensuring its continued relevance throughout various phases.

Prenatal and Postnatal Yoga:

Specifically address the adaptability of yoga during significant life events, such as pregnancy. Highlight the benefits of prenatal and postnatal yoga as a supportive practice that addresses the unique needs of individuals during these transformative periods.

4. Creating Personalized Routines:

Designing Home Practices:

Encourage the creation of personalized home practices. Providing guidance on designing routines that cater to individual preferences, time constraints, and comfort levels empowers individuals to integrate yoga seamlessly into their daily lives.

Incorporating Short Sessions:

Emphasize the effectiveness of short yoga sessions. Suggesting brief but consistent practices, such as 10-15 minutes per day, makes it more manageable for individuals to incorporate yoga into their routines.

5. Community Engagement and Support:

Participating in Group Classes:

Stress the value of community engagement through group classes. Whether in-person or virtual, participating in group sessions fosters a sense of connection, accountability, and shared motivation, enhancing the overall experience of yoga.

Joining Online Communities:

Recommend joining online yoga communities. Platforms, where individuals can share experiences, seek advice, celebrate milestones, create a virtual support network, and offer encouragement and inspiration.

6. Incorporating Yoga into Daily Rituals:

Morning or Evening Rituals:

Promote the incorporation of yoga into daily rituals. Suggest establishing a morning or evening routine that includes a brief yoga practice, making it an integral part of the day and reinforcing its importance in daily life.

Creating Sacred Spaces:

Encourage the creation of a sacred space for yoga practice. Designating a corner or room for yoga fosters a sense of dedication and mindfulness, enhancing the overall experience and motivation to continue the practice.

7. **Continual Learning and Exploration:**

Pursuing Advanced Training:

Highlight the option of pursuing advanced training in yoga. Whether through workshops, teacher training programs, or specialized courses, continual learning allows individuals to deepen their understanding, refine their practice, and stay inspired.

Exploring Workshops and Retreats:

Recommend attending workshops and yoga retreats. These immersive experiences offer opportunities for rejuvenation, learning from experienced instructors, and connecting with like-minded individuals, reigniting enthusiasm for the practice.

8. Mindful Integration into Daily Life:

Yoga Beyond the Mat:

Emphasize the concept of yoga extending beyond the mat. Encourage individuals to apply yogic principles to daily life, fostering mindfulness, gratitude, and compassion in various situations, thereby integrating the essence of yoga into their overall lifestyle.

Mindful Eating Practices:

Highlight mindful eating practices as an extension of yoga. Incorporating conscious eating habits aligns with the principles of mindfulness, promoting a holistic approach to well-being that extends beyond physical postures.

9. Celebrating Milestones and Progress:

Acknowledging Personal Growth:

Encourage individuals to acknowledge and celebrate their personal growth. Recognizing improvements in flexibility, strength, and emotional well-being serves as positive reinforcement, reinforcing the value of a continued yoga practice.

Maintaining a Yoga Journal:

Suggest maintaining a yoga journal. Recording personal reflections, achievements, and insights creates a tangible record of progress, fostering a sense of accomplishment and motivation to sustain the practice.

10. Teaching Yoga to Others:

Becoming a Yoga Instructor:

Explore the option of becoming a certified yoga instructor. For those deeply passionate about yoga, the journey may evolve into sharing the practice with others, creating a fulfilling and purposeful path that intertwines with ongoing personal practice.

Teaching Family and Friends:

Emphasize the joy of teaching yoga to family and friends. Introducing loved ones to the benefits of yoga creates a shared experience, deepening connections and establishing a support system that encourages everyone to continue their practice.

A Lifelong Journey of Transformation:

Conclude this section by emphasizing that yoga is a lifelong journey of transformation. Encourage individuals to view their practice not as a fleeting activity but as an ongoing exploration that evolves with them, offering continuous benefits for physical, mental, and spiritual well-being.

Embracing the Ever-Evolving Path:

Express the idea of embracing the ever-evolving path of yoga. As individuals navigate the various stages of life, the practice of yoga remains a constant companion, adapting, supporting, and enriching their journey toward holistic well-being.

By fostering a mindset of continuity, adaptability, and personalization, individuals can weave the practice of yoga seamlessly into the fabric of their lives, ensuring that its transformative benefits endure throughout the journey of self-discovery and well-being.

8.3 Inspiring Others: Spreading the Joy of Kids' Yoga

The transformative joy of kids' yoga is a gift worth sharing, not just for the well-being of children but as a ripple effect that enriches families, communities, and beyond. In this section, we explore ways to inspire and encourage others to embrace the joy of kids' yoga, fostering a collective movement towards mindful living, empowerment, and the holistic development of young minds.

1. **Sharing Personal Experiences:**

Expressing Personal Transformations:

Share personal experiences and transformations through kids' yoga. Whether as a parent, caregiver, or instructor, conveying the positive impact on your life or the lives of the children you work with adds authenticity and inspires others to explore the practice.

Narrating Joyful Moments:

Narrate joyful moments experienced during kids' yoga sessions. Illustrate how laughter, creativity, and a sense of accomplishment create an environment where children and adults alike thrive, fostering curiosity and a desire to join in the fun.

2. **Organizing Community Events:**

Yoga in the Park:

Organize community events that showcase the joy of kids' yoga. Events like "Yoga in the Park" or family-friendly yoga picnics create a welcoming space for families and community members to experience the benefits firsthand.

Collaborative Workshops:

Collaborate with local organizations to host workshops. Partnering with schools, community centers, or wellness organizations expands the reach of kids' yoga, introducing its joys to diverse audiences.

3.   Creating Engaging Content:

Online Tutorials and Demonstrations:

Produce online tutorials and demonstrations. Sharing accessible content on platforms like social media or YouTube provides a valuable resource for parents, caregivers, and educators interested in incorporating kids' yoga into their routines.

Inspiring Stories and Testimonials:

Feature inspiring stories and testimonials. Showcase the transformative journeys of children and families who have embraced kids' yoga, creating a collection of narratives that resonate with others contemplating the practice.

4.   Engaging Schools and Educational Institutions:

Integrating Yoga into School Curricula:

Advocate for the integration of yoga into school curricula. Highlight the academic and emotional benefits of kids' yoga to educators and administrators, fostering an understanding of how yoga contributes to a positive and focused learning environment.

Parent-Teacher Workshops:

Conduct parent-teacher workshops on the benefits of kids' yoga. Empower parents and educators with knowledge about how yoga enhances children's cognitive abilities, emotional regulation, and overall well-being.

5. Collaborating with Parenting Communities:

Parenting Blog Collaborations:

Collaborate with parenting bloggers. Contributing articles, guest posts, or interviews to parenting platforms allows for the dissemination of information about kids' yoga and its positive impact on family dynamics.

Parenting Community Events:

Participate in parenting community events. Engage with local parenting groups, playdates, or community gatherings to share insights, answer questions, and introduce parents to the joy of incorporating yoga into family life.

6. **Youth and Community Organizations:**

Youth Club Collaborations:

Collaborate with youth clubs and organizations. Engaging with local youth groups provides an opportunity to introduce kids' yoga in a fun and interactive way, fostering a sense of camaraderie and inclusivity.

Community Outreach Programs:

Organize community outreach programs. Partnering with organizations focused on child development, well-being, or community outreach allows for the broader dissemination of the benefits of kids' yoga to diverse populations.

7. **Social Media Campaigns:**

#KidsYogaJoy Campaign:

Launch a social media campaign, such as #KidsYogaJoy. Encourage participants to share photos, videos, and stories of the joy experienced in kids' yoga sessions, creating a digital movement that inspires others to join in.

Live Sessions and Challenges:

Conduct live yoga sessions and challenges. Utilize platforms like Instagram or Facebook to host live sessions, interactive challenges, or Q&A sessions, fostering a sense of community and enthusiasm for kids' yoga.

8. Collaborative Initiatives with Wellness Professionals:

Collaborating with Pediatricians and Therapists:

Collaborate with pediatricians and therapists. Engaging with healthcare professionals allows for the integration of kids' yoga as a complementary approach to physical and mental well-being, creating a bridge between medical and holistic practices.

Wellness Expos and Fairs:

Participate in wellness expos and fairs. Showcasing kids' yoga at community events dedicated to well-being introduces the practice to a diverse audience, fostering partnerships with wellness-oriented businesses and professionals.

9. School Holiday Programs:

Yoga-themed School Holiday Programs:

Propose yoga-themed school holiday programs. Offering specialized kids' yoga programs during school breaks provides parents with an enriching and fun option for their children, promoting the integration of yoga into family routines.

Parent-Child Yoga Workshops:

Organize parent-child yoga workshops. These interactive sessions create a bonding experience between parents and children, reinforcing the joy of practicing yoga together.

10. Showcasing the Diversity of Kids' Yoga:

Inclusive Representation in Marketing:

Ensure inclusive representation in marketing materials. Showcase the diversity of children participating in kids' yoga to emphasize its accessibility and relevance to children of all backgrounds, abilities, and family structures.

Highlighting Adaptive Practices:

Highlight adaptive practices for diverse needs. Showcase how kids' yoga can be adapted for children with special needs, fostering an inclusive approach that inspires instructors, parents, and caregivers to make yoga accessible to every child.

A Movement of Joy and Empowerment:

Conclude this section by envisioning a movement of joy and empowerment sparked by the spreading of kids' yoga. Emphasize that the collective efforts of individuals sharing their experiences, organizing events, and collaborating with various communities contribute to a culture where kids' yoga is celebrated and embraced.

Invitation to Join the Movement:

Extend an invitation for others to join the movement. Encourage everyone, whether parents, caregivers, educators, or wellness enthusiasts, to play a role in spreading the joy of kids' yoga, fostering a positive impact on the lives of children and communities.

By inspiring others and collectively spreading the joy of kids' yoga, we create a ripple effect of well-being, mindfulness, and empowerment that extends far beyond the mat. Each shared experience, every community event, and all collaborative initiatives contribute to a movement where the transformative power of kids' yoga becomes a shared celebration of growth, joy, and holistic development.

Conclusion

As we conclude our exploration into the world of "Yoga for Kids: The Ultimate Guide to Yoga for Bend, Breathe, and Grow with Empowering Children through Mindfulness, Flexibility, and Fun with Yoga," we find ourselves immersed in the transformative potential that kids' yoga offers. This guide serves as a compass, navigating the path toward the holistic development of children—physically, mentally, and emotionally.

Reflecting on the Journey:

Empowered Minds and Bodies:

Our journey through these pages has been a celebration of empowered minds and flexible bodies. The practices of kids' yoga, intricately woven with mindfulness, flexibility, and fun, have become the tools for children to navigate the challenges of growing up with resilience and joy.

A Tapestry of Positivity:

The narrative unfolds as a tapestry of positivity, illustrating the myriad ways in which yoga becomes a companion in fostering self-discovery, emotional well-being, and a sense of community. From the basics to advanced poses, from mindful breathing to creative expression, every aspect contributes to the rich and vibrant fabric of kids' yoga.

Key Takeaways from Our Guide:

The Essence of Yoga Defined:

We delved into the very essence of yoga, understanding it not merely as a physical practice but as a holistic journey encompassing the mind, body, and spirit. Through detailed explanations of poses, breathing techniques, and mindfulness practices, we demystified yoga, making it accessible and enjoyable for children.

Building Foundations and Beyond:

Chapter by chapter, we explored the foundational principles of kids' yoga, from understanding its benefits to guiding children through poses. We emphasized the importance of adaptability, meeting children where they are, and creating an environment where each child feels seen, heard, and empowered.

Mindfulness as a Lifelong Skill:

Mindfulness emerged as a guiding thread throughout, underscoring its importance as a lifelong skill. Beyond the physical postures, mindfulness became the anchor, empowering children to face challenges with clarity, resilience, and a deep sense of presence.

The Evolution of Practice:

From Gentle Poses to Advanced Asanas:

The journey took us through gentle poses for beginners, intermediate postures for growing bodies, and advanced asanas for building strength and focus. With each progression, children not only honed their physical abilities but also cultivated a mindset of perseverance and self-discovery.

Breathing Techniques and Mindfulness Integration:

The exploration of breathing techniques and mindfulness practices further enriched the practice of kids' yoga. Breath became a powerful tool for stress relief, and mindfulness became the lens through which children experienced a deeper connection to themselves and the world around them.

Fostering Joy and Connection:

Making Yoga Fun:

We discovered the importance of making yoga fun, weaving creative games, music, and partner activities into the fabric of practice. The integration of joy became a catalyst, fostering a love for movement and self-expression that extends far beyond the mat.

Community and Support:

Emphasizing the role of community, we explored how kids' yoga extends beyond individual practice. The shared experiences, the collaborative initiatives, and the support networks formed contribute to a sense of belonging and encouragement for both children and those guiding them.

Overcoming Challenges and Looking Ahead:

Addressing Concerns and Adapting Practices:

Acknowledging challenges, we navigated through common concerns in kids' yoga, adapting practices for different needs and circumstances. The guide became a resource for overcoming obstacles, ensuring that yoga remains inclusive and beneficial for all children.

Building a Supportive Community:

We delved into the importance of building a supportive community, recognizing that the journey of kids' yoga is not solitary but one that thrives on collective wisdom, shared joys, and mutual encouragement.

A Lifelong Journey of Well-Being:

Lifelong Benefits Unveiled:

Unveiling the lifelong benefits of kids' yoga, we explored how its impact transcends childhood. From physical well-being to emotional resilience, the practices learned in kids' yoga become enduring companions, shaping individuals into mindful, adaptable, and balanced adults.

Encouraging a Continued Yoga Practice:

The guide concluded by encouraging a continued yoga practice, providing insights on setting realistic goals, adapting to life changes, and weaving yoga into daily routines. The emphasis was on yoga as a lifelong journey, a dynamic and personal exploration that evolves with individuals throughout their lives.

Spreading the Joy:

Inspiring Others to Join the Movement:

Finally, we explored the joy of spreading kids' yoga beyond the individual practice. Through personal experiences, community events, online content, and collaborative initiatives, we envisioned a movement that inspires others to embrace the transformative joy of kids' yoga.

Invitation to Join the Journey:

The conclusion extends an invitation for others to join this movement of joy and empowerment. It envisions a collective celebration where the benefits of kids' yoga ripple through families, communities, and beyond, creating a culture of well-being, mindfulness, and growth.

In essence, "Yoga for Kids" is not just a guide; it is an invitation to embark on a journey—one that bends with flexibility, breathes with mindfulness, and grows with the empowering spirit of children. As we close this chapter, may the practices and insights shared within these pages continue to unfold, inspiring a world where every child has the opportunity to bend, breathe, and grow with the transformative joy of yoga.

www.ingramcontent.com/pod-product-compliance
Lightning Source LLC
Chambersburg PA
CBHW080926260726
48661CB00010B/3812